AF553675

# Integrated Livestock Farming Systems

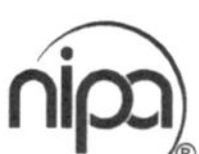

NIPA® GENX ELECTRONIC RESOURCES & SOLUTIONS P. LTD.
New Delhi-110 034

## About the Authors

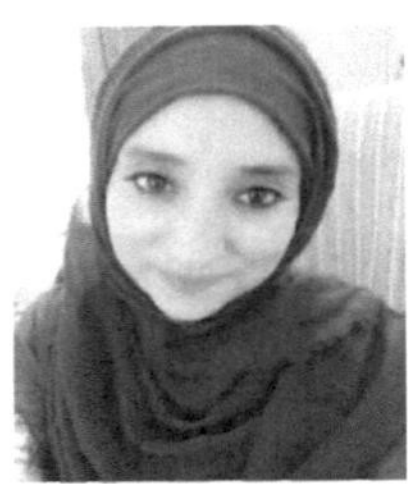

**Dr. Hina Ashraf Waiz** received a Bachelor of Veterinary Sciences degree from Nanaji Deshmukh Veterinary University in Jabalpur, Madhya Pradesh, India. MV.Sc in Livestock Production Management with a specialization in Poultry from the Sher-Kashmir University of Agriculture Sciences & Technology, Kashmir and a Ph.D. in Livestock Production Management from the Rajasthan University of Veterinary & Animal Science Bikaner, India. She is currently employed as an Assistant Professor in the Department of Livestock Production Management at the College of Veterinary and Animal Science, Udaipur Campus (Rajasthan University of Veterinary & Animal Science- Bikaner, India). She previously held the position of Assistant Professor in the Department of Animal Production at Wollo University in Dessie, Ethiopia. Dr. Hina Ashraf Waiz, helped students in designing different animal house models for livestock and strengthened the LPM laboratory. She has prepared more than 8 laboratory manuals for B.V.Sc students and published more than 22 research articles in various national and international journals, 25 research abstracts and various book chapters. She is the member of ISAPM (Indian Society of Animal Production Management).She has guided 3 M.V.Sc students. Her contributions have been recognized through a number of awards, including the Best Faculty of the Year Award in 2011 for significant contributions to undergrad teaching, the Best Research Paper Award in 2018 at a national conference from the Society of Veterinary Biotechnology, the Gold Medal in 2021 for Excellence in Research from the Journal of Global Management, and the National Best Scientist Award -2022 in Animal Husbandry & Veterinary Sciences from the International Multidisciplinary Research Foundation, Hyderabad.

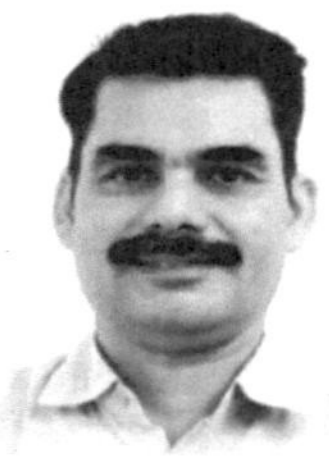

**Dr. Lokesh Gautam** received a Bachelor of Veterinary Sciences degree, MV.Sc, and a Ph.D. in Animal Genetics and Breeding with a specialization in Animal Breeding from the Rajasthan University of Veterinary & Animal Science Bikaner, India. He is currently working as an Assistant Professor in the Department of Animal Genetics and Breeding at the College of Veterinary and Animal Science, Udaipur Campus (Rajasthan University of Veterinary & Animal Science- Bikaner, India).He has prepared more than 7 laboratory manuals for B.V.Sc students and published more than 20 research articles in various national and international journals, 26 research abstracts and various book chapters. He is the life member of ISAPM (Indian Society of Animal Production Management) and ISSGPU (Indian Society for Sheep and Goat Production &Utilization).He has guided 1 M.V.Sc students. He has served as project in-charge and co-incharge for a number of projects, including the Malvi Cattle Breeding Farm in Jhalawar, Rajasthan, the RACP for goats (a World Bank project), and currently Project in-charge, MSSP- ICAR (Mega Sheep

Seed Project) for Sonadi sheep at the College of Veterinary and Animal Science in Navania, Udaipur. His contributions have been honored with a number of awards, including a gold medal in 2003 and 2018 for his post-graduate and PhD work, as well as a vice chancellors award in 2022 for effective farm management.

# Integrated Livestock Farming Systems

**Hina Ashraf Waiz**
B.V.Sc & A.H, M.V.Sc & PhD.
Assistant Professor
Department of Livestock Production and Management
College of Veterinary and Animal Sciences, Navania, Udaipur
Rajasthan University of Veterinary & Animal Sciences
Bikaner- 334001, Rajasthan

**Lokesh Gautam**
Assistant Professor
Department of Animal Genetics & Breeding (AGB)
College of Veterinary and Animal Science, Navania, Udaipur
Rajasthan University of Veterinary and Animal Sciences
Bikaner- 334001, Rajasthan

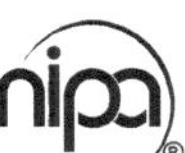

**NIPA® GENX ELECTRONIC RESOURCES & SOLUTIONS P. LTD.**
New Delhi-110 034

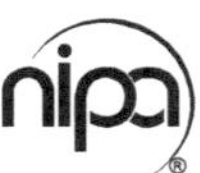

**NIPA® GENX ELECTRONIC RESOURCES & SOLUTIONS P. LTD.**

101,103, Vikas Surya Plaza, CU Block
L.S.C. Market, Pitam Pura, New Delhi-110 034
Ph : +91 11 27341616, 27341717, 27341718
E-mail: newindiapublishingagency@gmail.com
Website: www.nipabooks.com
***For customer assistance, please contact***
Phone: + 91-11-27 34 17 17
Fax: + 91-11-27 34 16 16
E-Mail: feedbacks@nipabooks.com



ISBN: 978-81-19103-16-4



Composed and Designed by NIPA®.

# Preface

The main goal of developing this book was to create a simplified handbook on integrated livestock farming for PG. & Ph.D. scholars, farmers and entrepreneurs. This handbook has all the information need to set up any size or type of integrated livestock unit. The ILFS aims to promote agriculture holistically by integrating animal husbandry and other fundamental agricultural practice-related activities. It has the potential to turn the enterprise profitable. The government plans to implement a seven-point strategy, which includes boosting productivity, making efficient use of input costs, lowering post-harvest losses, adding value, and reforming agriculture marketing, to double farmers' incomes over the next five years. This handbook will enhance knowledge and expertise of the farmers and entrepreneurs already in ILFS model or wish to set up an ILFS model. Anyone with desire and initiative may start a successful and profitable enterprise by following the detailed advice, guidelines, and suggestions in this book.

Finally we express gratitude to our family members for their constant support and encouragement. We also want to express our sincere thanks to NIPA Genx Electronic Resources And Solutions Pvt. Ltd., New Delhi for publishing this book.

**Hina Ashraf Waiz**
**Lokesh Gautam**

# Contents

# 1

# Introduction

*Hina Ashraf Waiz*

The large and diverse livestock resources of India benefit millions of people in rural areas, enhancing their standard of living. The key elements of sustainable agriculture are livestock resources. India has a population of 535.78 million livestock. According to $20^{th}$ livestock census 2019,India ranks first in the world for the number of buffalo (109.85 million), second in number of cattle (192.49 million), third for the number of sheep (74.26 million), fifth for the number of chickens and ducks (851.81 million), and tenth for the number of camels (2.5 lakhs). About 8.8% of India's population is engaged by the livestock industry, which provides a living for two-thirds of the country's rural communities. About 8.8% of India's population is engaged by the livestock industry, which provides a living for two-thirds of the country's rural communities (Dash, 2017). The livestock sector contributes 4.11% GDP (Gross DomesticProduction) and 25.6% of total Agriculture GDP. India is number one milk producer in the world with 176.3 million tons of milk. Similarly it is producing about 95.2 billion of eggs, 41.5 million kg of wool and 7.7 million tons of meat annually (Singh, 2018). Additionally, the livestock helps to produce valuable manure, leather, and pelts.

Small and marginal farmers in rural India have a long history of using integrated livestock farming systems. For farmers to earn more money, crop-based agriculture must be diversified to include dairy, goatery, fishing, poultry, duckery, and other enterprises (Ray et al., 2012).Small and marginal farmers represent the majority of the farming community in India (85%), although they only possess 44% of the country's total arable land. Indian agriculture is labor-intensive and requires a lot of manpower and energy, but despite their efforts especially those of small and marginal farmers are still unable to make a living (Sahoo et al., 2015). This is because they have to pay for all of their inputs, including seeds, livestock, fertilizer, pesticides, energy, feed, and labor Consideration should be given to integrated farming systems in order to meet the basic needs of these farm families, including food (cereal, pulses, oilseeds, milk, fruit, honey, meat, etc.), feed fodder, fibre, and fuel (IFS). The farming system puts a significant amount of emphasis on effectively recycling farm wastes. In an integrated farming system, several farming system components collaborate to achieve a greater overall productivity than the sum of their individual outputs. The efficiency of resource utilization is increased when the output from one enterprise becomes the input for another. Farmers' land holdings are fragmented, therefore it's important to include land-based businesses like fisheries, poultry, apiaries, field crops, and horticulture into the bio-physical and socio-economic conditions of the farmers to increase farmer's profitability and dependability (Behera et al., 2004). Through the sale of milk, the livestock sector gives farmers a consistent source of income and employment during hard situation. In times of adversity, livestock serves as a moving bank and an asset that gives farmers financial security. In addition to serving as a critical supply of protein for human consumption, livestock also acts as a source of money, insurance against crop production hazards, and a coping mechanism for shocks to one's way of life. Agriculture provides seasonal employment for five to six months out of the year, and livestock husbandry provides employment during the lean season. Farmers can also rely on milk, meat, and eggs from the livestock industry for their nutritional security. Owning top livestock, such as pedigreed bulls and high-yielding dairy cows, provides farmers a sense of self-worth. Cow dung and other waste products from the fodder industry break down to produce excellent farmyard manure.

The small and marginal farmers depend upon bullocks for ploughing, carting and transport of both inputs and outputs. The bullocks are saving a lot of fuel which is necessary input for using mechanical power operations. Draught animal power is listed as one of the 14 renewable energy sources at the UN Conference on New and Renewable Sources of Energy in Nairobi because of its economic significance (Ramaswamy, 1998). In steep terrain, pack animals including camels, horses, donkeys, ponies, mules, and mithun help move products between different regions of the nation. Numerous locations use livestock as a biological weed controller for various crops. By boosting family income and creating gainful employment, livestock contributes significantly to the economic development of rural areas, especially for women, smallholders, and marginal farmers who lack access to land.

**Table 1:** Trends in Livestock population (Millions)

| **Species** | **1951** | **1982** | **1992** | **2003** | **2007** | **2012** | **2019** |
|---|---|---|---|---|---|---|---|
| Cattle | 155.3 | 192.5 | 204.6 | 185.2 | 199.1 | 190.9 | 192.49 |
| Buffalo | 43.4 | 69.8 | 84.2 | 97.9 | 105.3 | 108.7 | 109.85 |
| **Total Bovines** | **198.7** | **262.4** | **289.0** | **283.1** | **304.4** | **300.0** | **302.79** |
| Sheep | 39.1 | 48.8 | 50.8 | 61.5 | 71.6 | 65.1 | 74.26 |
| Goat | 47.2 | 95.3 | 115.3 | 124.4 | 140.5 | 135.2 | 148.88 |
| Horses & ponies | 1.5 | 0.9 | 0.8 | 0.8 | 0.6 | 0.6 | 3.4 |
| Camels | 0.6 | 1.1 | 1.0 | 0.6 | 0.5 | 0.4 | 2.5 |
| Pigs | 4.4 | 10.1 | 12.8 | 13.5 | 11.1 | 10.3 | 9.0 |
| Mules | 0.1 | 0.1 | 0.2 | 0.2 | 0.1 | 0.2 | 0.8 |
| Donkeys | 1.3 | 1.0 | 1.0 | 0.7 | 0.4 | 0.3 | 0.1 |
| Yaks | - | 0.1 | 0.1 | 0.1 | 0.1 | 0.1 | 0.5 |
| **Total livestock** | **292.8** | **419.6** | **470.9** | **485.0** | **529.7** | **512.1** | **535.78** |
| Poultry | 73.5 | 207.7 | 307.1 | 489.0 | 648.8 | 729.2 | 851.81 |

(*Source*: Department of Animal Husbandry, Dairying and Fisheries)

**Table 2:** Trend in production of milk, eggs, meat and wool in India

| Year | Milk (Million Tones) | Eggs(Billion Nos) | Meat(Million Tons) | Wool (Million kgs) |
|---|---|---|---|---|
| 2010-11 | 121.8 | 63.0 | 5.49 | 43.0 |
| 2011-12 | 127.9 | 66.5 | 5.51 | 44.7 |
| 2012-13 | 132.4 | 69.7 | 5.95 | 46.1 |
| 2013-14 | 137.7 | 74.8 | 6.24 | 47.9 |
| 2014-15 | 146.3 | 78.5 | 6.69 | 48.1 |
| 2015-16 | 155.49 | 82.93 | 7.02 | 43.58 |
| 2016-17 | 165.40 | 88.14 | 7.39 | 43.54 |
| 2017-18 | 176.35 | 95.22 | 7.66 | 41.46 |
| 2018-19 | 187.75 | 103.80 | 8.11 | 40.42 |
| 2019-20 | 198.44 | 114.38 | 8.60 | 36.76 |
| 2020-21 | 209.96 | 122.05 | 8.80 | 36.93 |

(*Source*: Department of Animal Husbandry, Dairying and Fisheries)

# 2

# Farming System

*Hina Ashraf Waiz*

A farming system is composed of several farm activities, such as cropping systems, horticulture, livestock, fisheries, forestry, and poultry, as well as the tools the farmer has at his disposal to raise these things profitably. However, a lot of definitions generally express the same concept, which is that it is a technique to achieve profitable and sustainable agricultural production in order to meet the varied needs of the farming community while sparing the natural resource base and environmental quality. Definitions that are relatively new include:

According to Pandey et al. (1992), ''The farming system is a collection of agricultural operations like crops, livestock, aquaculture, agroforestry, and fruit crops to which farm families devote their resources in order to effectively manage the surrounding environment for the accomplishment of family objectives''.

The term "farming system" refers to a profitable arrangement of agricultural operations (cropping systems, horticulture, livestock, fishing, forestry, and poultry) and the tools at the farmer's disposal to raise them. It effectively interacts with the environment without upsetting the ecological and socioeconomic balance while still attempting to achieve the country's objectives (Jayanthi et al., 2000).

In general, a farming system (whole farm business) consists of three key elements: **(i)** the crop component (cereals, pulses, oilseeds, sugar, fibre, vegetable, fruits, agroforestry, etc.); **(ii)** the animal component (cattle, goats, sheep, etc.); and **(iii)** homestead farming (biogas, post-harvest, value-added products, grinding, splitting of pulses), which also includes other related activities carried out with Each of the aforementioned elements could include one or more different activities or processes (Rana, 2015).

## Farming system research (FSR)

The Farming system research (FSR) should be farmer-centered, system-oriented, problem-solving, inter-disciplinary, and designed to supplement traditional disciplinary research. Farming system research should test new technology through field trials and give farmers feedback. An alternative to the "**Transfer of Technology**" paradigm (TOT) is the **"Farmer First and Last"** (FFL) model, which is based on the farmer's priorities and perceptions rather than the scientist's professional preferences.

## Classification of farming system based on income, value of products or comparative advantages

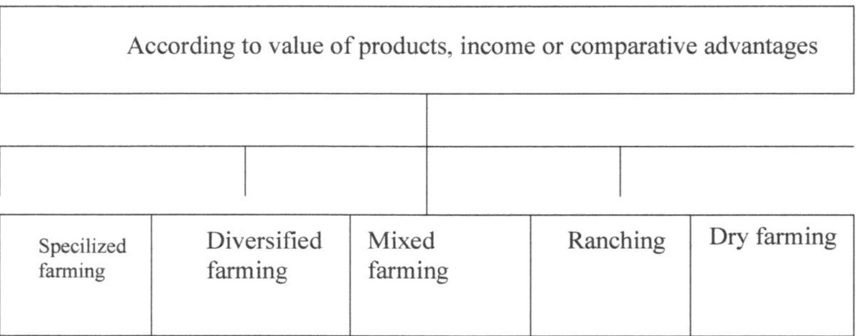


**1. Specialized farming:** The term "specialist farm" refers to a farm where at least 50% of the farm's revenue comes from a single enterprise, such as crops, cattle, dairy products, poultry, etc.

## Advantages

- **Better Land Use:** Growing crops on land that is best suited for specialty streams is more advantageous.
- **Better Marketing:** It provides better marketing options because it makes it possible to grade, process, store, transport, and finance the goods.
- **Less Labor and Equipment Needed:** Specialized farming typically doesn't call for highly skilled people or specialized machinery.
- **Enhanced Productivity & Skill of the Labor:** Specialization enables a worker to be more productive and skillful at carrying out a certain range of tasks.
- **Simple Maintenance:** Because specialized farming concentrates more on a specific task, farm records are easy to maintain.

- **Large Output:** High production intensity leads to a comparatively large amount of output.
- **Better Management:** With fewer enterprises to supervise on the farm, it will be easier to identify and get rid of waste sources.

**Disadvantages**

- **Seasonal Less Demand:** There is less demand for a product when a harvest fails and the market price of the commodity declines.
- **Lack of Soil Fertility:** Without crop rotation, it is impossible to keep the soil fertile.
- **Income irregularity:** Because payments are only made once or twice a year, the farm's income is erratic.
- **Inefficient Resource Utilization:** In contrast to diversified farming, which places emphasis on a variety of areas, productive resources including land, labor, and capital are underutilized.
- **Knowledge of Other Activities:** Due to the extreme specialization of any given activity, knowledge of other enterprises is irrelevant.
- Farm byproducts cannot be properly utilized due to a shortage of livestock on the farm.
- The common knowledge of farm businesses gets constrained.

**Mixed farming:** A mixed farming operation combines the raising of livestock and the production of crops. To create a balanced and effective farming system, the livestock enterprises (cows, buffaloes, sheep, goats, and fisheries) complement crop production. In mixed farming, livestock activities must provide at least 10% of the gross income. Under Indian conditions, the maximum is 49%. Therefore, a mixed farm is one that derives at least 10 to 49% of its income from livestock. In mixed farming, crop production includes cows and buffaloes.

**Advantages**

- Due to the proper use of farm byproducts, it provides the maximum return on investment.
- It offers employment all year round.
- Effective use of equipment, labor, land, and other resources.
- The crop's byproducts, such as straw, hay, and fodder, are fed to livestock, which in turn produce milk.

- Livestock manures help to keep the soil fertile.
- It assists in meeting all of the family members' food needs.
- It is feasible to cultivate intensively.
- A person can support his family if one source of income is lost by having another one.
- Draft animals for farming and rural transportation include milk cow.
- Mixed farming raises a farmer's social standing.
- Because animal power is the primary source of power in agriculture, livestock and agriculture are very tightly related in India. In such situations, mixed farming will work best for Indian settings.
- FYM is the key source for preserving soil fertility.
- Animals make good use of subsidiary and by-products on farms and offer milk as a result.

## Disadvantages

- Indigenous cultivation techniques are still in use today.
- When draught and milch animals are unable to produce, they should be sold.
- To replace aged animals, a healthy calf should be raised.

## Required of Mixed Farming

i) Complicated management practices.

ii) Sound cropping scheme.

iii) Good cattle in suitable number.

iv) Transport facility.

v) Marketing facilities

**3. Ranching:** In contrast to other types of agricultural and livestock production, a ranch allows its livestock to graze on the natural vegetation. Crop production or tilling are not done on ranch land. The ranchers use the public grazing property because they don't own any land of their own. One or more operators spend the most of their time as ranchers. Australia, America, Tibet, and some regions of India use ranching. In contrast to other types of agricultural and livestock production, a ranch allows its livestock to graze on the natural vegetation. Crop production or tilling is not done on ranch land. The ranchers use the public grazing property because they don't own any land of their own. One or more operators spend the most of their time as ranchers. Australia, America, Tibet, and some regions of India use ranching.

**4. Dry farming: Farmers** on dry areas who receive 750 mm or even less of rainfall struggle to earn a living. The main issue with farm management in these tracts is the retention of soil moisture for crops that are completely dependent on rainfall. The following practices must be adopted in dry farming:

a) Timely preparing the land in a position where it can best absorb and hold onto the moisture that is available.

b) Timing and appropriate inter-culturing throughout the crop's growth.

c) Increasing the soil's ability to hold water by profitably applying organic manure.

d) Making use of tools that can quickly break through the soil's surface.

e) Construction of fields.

f) Using the best seed rates.

g) Controlling overpopulations of plants.

h) Mixing crops.

## What is integrated farming?

A subset of farming system research (FSR) study is called integrated farming systems (IFS). An integrated farming system is an environmentally beneficial method that maximizes the use of farm resources by converting waste from one enterprise into nutrients for another. The efficient use of land, labor, and other resources within a farm family is achieved through the scientific integration of several interdependent and interacting farm enterprises, which provides year-round income to farmers specifically located in the handicapped zone. Keep poultry in the top layer, for instance, and use their manure. The lowest strata are habitat to pigs, and the remaining pond water is used for agriculture and fodder crops. Utilizing integrated farming techniques, emissions can be recycled as fertilizer for orchards and feed crops.

According to Panke et al. (2010), integration is designed to ensure that the output of one enterprise or component becomes the input for the other enterprises, resulting in a high degree of complementary effects. The goal of IFS is to reduce waste from the various farm subsystems, which enhances rural households' access to work, nutritional security, and income.

## Difference between mixed farming and integrated farming

An integrated farming system involves interdependent and mutually beneficial activities. Contrarily, mixed farming systems include coexisting, autonomous components like crops and livestock.

Crops and cattle are often combined in mixed farming; however this practice has little to do with resource conservation. While in an integrated agricultural system, crops and livestock work together to generate a synergy, and recycling enables the best possible use of the resources that are available. Animal production and processing can increase agricultural productivity by increasing nutrients that improve soil fertility and lowering the need for artificial fertilizers, while crop residues can be utilized as animal feed.

## Need for Integrated Farming

- **Shrinkage in arable land:** Area under crops is getting smaller every day as a result of urbanization, industry, population growth, and the building of structures and highways. As a result, the carrying capacity of the land per unit of capital has drastically decreased. India's population is projected to be 137 and 166 cores in 2030 and 2050 AD, respectively, but its arable land will decrease to 141.3 and 131.3 million hectares (Tripathi et al. 2011).

- **Small and irregular holding:** The average holding of a farm has been declining, and more than 80% of operational farms in India are smaller than 1 hectare.

- **Seasonality in work, income, and migration:** Only four months of the wet season are permitted for harvesting in areas which are fed with rain. Employment prospects are sparse during other seasons. As a result, a lot of men who are farmers move to the metropolis in search of work. Year-round employment possibilities in rural areas are required to deter migration.

- **Decline in resource base:** Long-term human population preservation is the ultimate goal of sustainable agriculture. Identifying the most effective method of employing internal inputs for long-term livestock and crop production that generates a positive return on investment is the optimal way to accomplish this.

- **Household requirement:** To achieve food and nutritional security, a state or country must ensure that every one of its citizens has access to a minimum quality variety of food items, such as a sufficient and balanced diet. In order to meet all of a household's needs, small and marginal farmers who produce timber are also essential.

## Principles of Integrative Farming System

- A sufficient quantity of high-quality food, fibre, fodder, and industrial raw materials should be generated.
- The system must accommodate societal demands.
- The system should continue to run a successful farming operation.
- The system should ensure that the sustainability of natural resources and that the environment is protected.

## The factors affecting the adoption of the Integrated Farming System

- The region's soil and climate characteristics.
- The accessibility of resources, labor, and capital.
- Current proportion of resources that are being used.
- The planned integrated farming system's economics.
- Farmer's managerial abilities.

## Factors affecting the size and type of enterprises in an integrated farming system

- Farm size marketing resources available
- Climate of the region Technology availability and access
- soil quality and soil type
- Credit achievements (government aid)
- knowledge and expertise of farmers

## Integrated Livestock Farming System (ILFS)

In integrated farming system, agriculture can be combined with maintenance of fish, poultry, and cattle in one location to create year-round employment and earn additional money. The integrated livestock farming system (ILFS), which combines several farming methods with livestock, aids in the efficient use of natural resources, wastes/organic residues, and bio resource recycling.

For instance, a by-product of the rice crop known as paddy straw can be utilized as a good input for the production of mushrooms or as a source of dry feed for dairy animals. Similar to how dairy by-products like manure may be utilized as fish feed or as raw material for vermin-compost units, waste from mushroom cultivation (used straw) can be used as a raw material in compost or vermin-compost pits.

## Importance of Integrated Livestock Farming System (ILFS)

The integrated livestock farming system is based on idea that **"there is no waste"** and that **"waste is merely a misdirected resource that may be turned into another usable material for another purpose"** is the foundation of an integrated livestock production system. It is a method for effectively utilizing waste produced by various farming methods and helps farmers achieve self-sufficiency and independence. The majority of farmers currently have small, fragmented land holdings (less than 1 ha), and the area under agricultural cultivation is also getting smaller every day, which lowers the production of various crops. In agricultural operations, crop cultivation and harvesting are dependent on the season, and farmers are free at other times of the year. In this situation, integrating the livestock sector with various farming systems can provide year-round income and employment while also meeting the needs of farmers with small land holdings.

## Classification of Livestock -based Farming System

Farmers can use a variety of methods, as briefly described below, to implement ILFS in order to make better use of their landholdings and create a year-round source of sustainable revenue. This may include combinations such as :

1. Livestock-crop based farming system
2. Crop -livestock -fishery based farming system
3. Backyard poultry based farming system with crops and livestock
4. Crop –livestock- poultry -fishery farming system
5. Poultry-fish based farming system
6. Duck-Fish based farming system
7. Crop- livestock –fishery- biogas/vermicomposting system
8. Silvi-pastoral based farming system with small ruminant
9. Pig-fish based farming system
10. Rabbit-fish based farming system

### 1. Livestock -crop based farming system

Adoption combination possibilities include:

- **Agriculture-Horticulture-Cattle-Goat-Sheep agricultural system**
- **Dairy-vegetable-fodder agricultural system.**

It is the most popular farming system and is employed in the most parts of India. While livestock manure can boost agricultural output by enhancing soil fertility and supplementing minerals that reduce the usage of artificial fertilizers, agricultural crop leftovers can be used to feed animals in integrated crop livestock farming systems. Animals play important and varied functions in the operation of the farm, and not just because they produce livestock products (meat, milk, eggs, wool, and hides) or can be quickly turned into cash when needed. Animals convert plant energy into usable activity that may be done, such as transport, milling, logging, road construction, marketing, and lifting water for irrigation. Animal power is also utilized for ploughing and other tasks like these. Manure and other kinds of animal waste are also provided by animals. Animal waste plays two key functions in the system's overall sustainability:

**Enhancing nutrient cycling:** Organic matter and other elements found in excreta, such as nitrogen, phosphorus, and potassium, are crucial for sustaining soil fertility and structure. Its application boosts output while lowering the chance of soil deterioration.

**Providing energy**: The production of biogas and energy for use in homes (such as cooking and lighting) or rural industry begins with excreta (e.g. powering mills and water pumps). Biogas or dung cakes can be used as fuel in place of charcoal and wood.

Crop residues and other products that would normally provide a significant waste disposal issue can be fed to livestock as food, which is one of the main benefits of crop-livestock production systems. For instance, straw, spoiled fruits, grains, and household refuse can all be fed to animals. After being properly decomposed, the nearly 4,000–5,000 kg of dung and 3,500–4,000 lts of urine that a healthy cow excretes each year can be used as manure to fertilize fields instead of artificial fertilizers. Cow dung helps in the overall sustainability of the farming system (Godi et al. 2013).

Biogas is produced by using cow manure. Biogas is the source of renewable, alternative and sustainable energy with a ton of manure containing 8 kg of nitrogen, 4 kg of phosphorus, and 16 kg of potassium, manure is an excellent fertilizer. In addition to fertilizing the soil, manure additions enhance its cellular makeup and water-retentive abilities (Alam et al., 2000). On farm, nutrients can be recycled more effectively when animals and crops are integrated. The expense of weed control can be significantly decreased, often by as much as 40%, in areas where cattle are utilized to graze the vegetation around plantations of coconut, oil palm, and rubber. Animal draught is frequently utilized for farming, transportation, water hauling, and powering equipment for food preparation. According to Venkatakdari et al., (2008), dairy developed areas had 98% less farmer suicide complaints than commercial agricultural areas. Six buffalos were utilized for integrated farming, which increased employment from 400 to 904 man-days.

## 2. Crop livestock fishery based farming system

The components of livestock and fisheries can be merged as follows under this distinct crop:

- **Crop-Goat/Cow/Fish farming scheme**
- **System for cultivating crops, Azolla, cattle, and fish**

After harvesting the rice crop, the crop leftover, or paddy straw, can be given to cattle. By making more nitrogen and phosphorus available in the soil, livestock dung can be applied to agricultural fields to increase soil fertility. However, rice fields can also contribute to fish productivity because they provide fish's superior planktonic, periphytic, and benthic food. Fish are raised in the livestock plus crop farming system without any additional feed, using the animal dung that is already present to promote the growth of phytoplankton and zooplankton. In an integrated system, fishes like rohu, catla, mrigal, grass carp, common carp, and silver carp are well adapted.

Fish fingerlings may be stocked at rates ranging from 8000 to 8500 per hectare. For higher fish yields under integrated farming systems, a species ratio of 40% surface feeders (Silver carp and catla), 20% column feeders (rohu), 20 to 30% bottom feeders (common carp and mrigal), and 10 to 20% macro vegetation feeders (grass carp) is preferable.

## 3. Backyard poultry based farming system with crops and livestock

The integration of livestock with crops and backyard poultry farming can increase farmer incomes and improve food security. Sheep, goats, pigs, and poultry from the family's backyard serve as emergency sources of income. Birds scavenge on both the unprocessed grains in dung and the field wastes left over from threshing. Backyard poultry also existed before the insects and pests that cause diseases to spread among crops. It's not necessary to use separate inputs to provide the birds with more food. The farm family can get good sources of protein from eggs and chicken, which also regularly generates income.

As a result of scientific intervention, backyard poultry enhanced household income. Farm revenue was substituted as a secondary source of income by backyard poultry. The majority of women (51%) relied on backyard poultry for 6–10% of overall household income. Possessing high income (11–20%) from 28% of women, and only 7 women members had earnings from poultry of between 21 and 30 percent (Nirmala et al. 2012).

**4. Crop livestock poultry fishery farming system**

Farming system includes poultry, fisheries, and horticulture.

To lower the cost of fertilizers and feeds in fish farming, a duck, pig, poultry, and fish farming system can be combined. It is possible to raise chicken close to or over fish ponds, where the waste from the poultry will drop into the fish pond and be recycled. In an integrated farming two-tier housing system, the lower floor can be used for pigs over a fish pond and the top floor for poultry rearing. Excreta from poultry are used by pigs, and excreta from pigs are used by fish. This recycling of resources occurs because it promotes the growth of zooplankton and phytoplankton, which are consumed by fish.

**5. Poultry-fish based farming system**

To cut expenditures on fertilizers and feeds in fish culture and optimize benefits, poultry rearing for meat (broilers) or eggs (layers) can be combined with fish culture. Raising poultry over or close to the ponds is one option, and the waste from the birds can be recycled to fertilize the fishponds. When built above the water line using bamboo poles, poultry housing would directly fertilize fish ponds. The ideal birds for fish poultry integration are those kept in an intensive system. Birds are housed in small spaces with no access to the outside world. This kind of farming is best adapted to deep litter. It only need a 6 to 8 cm thick layer made of groundnut shells, sawdust, dry leaves, or chopped straw.

In the form of fully built up deep litter, poultry dung contains 3% nitrogen, 2% phosphate, and 2% potash. As a result, it functions as a good fertilizer that aids in the production of phytoplankton and zooplankton, which are used as fish feed in fish ponds. Therefore, adding more fertilizer to a fish pond to raise fish is not necessary. By doing this, fish production costs are reduced by 60%. Based on the fact that 25–30 birds may create 1 ton of dip litter per year, 500–600 birds are sufficient to fertilize a water spread area of 1 hectare for good fish productivity (Korikantimath et al., 2008).

**6. Duck-Fish based farming system**

A fish pond, which is a semi-closed biological system with a variety of aquatic animals and plants, offers ducks a great environment free of sickness. Ducks eat young frogs, tadpoles, and dragonflies in exchange, creating a safe environment for fish. Duck excrement directly enters the pond, providing vital minerals to promote the growth of natural food. This provides the benefits of homogenous fertilization and no energy loss. West Bengal, Assam, Kerala, Tamil Nadu, Andhra Pradesh, Bihar, Orissa, Tripura, and Karnataka are among the states that practice integrated farming. The "Indian runners" breed is the one that is most frequently employed in this system in India.

Due to the significant increase in fish and duck protein production per unit area, it is extremely profitable. Ducks are referred to as **"living manuring machines**." The duck poop is composed of 25% organic and 20% inorganic materials, including a variety of elements like carbon, phosphorus, potassium, nitrogen, calcium, etc. (Mahajan et al., 2012). As a result, it makes for an excellent supply of fertilizer in fish ponds for the growth of organisms that become fish food. Along with manuring, ducks also get rid of unwanted insects, snails, and their larvae, which could be the carriers of dangerous fish species and waterborne diseases that can infect humans. Additionally, ducks contribute to the release of nutrients from pond soil, especially when they stir up the pond's shoreline.

Ducks may occasionally be permitted to roam freely or may be placed in screened resting areas above the water for duck-fish culture. To provide uniform manuring, floating pens or huts made of bamboo splits may be suspended in the pond. These sheds can accommodate 15 to 20 ducks per square meter of space. The ducks should only be kept in ponds until they are big enough to be sold. Ducks may need to be replaced every two to three months, depending on their pace of growth. The typical selection age for ducklings is between 15 and 20 days. Depending on how long the fish are being cultured for and the amount of manure needed, the number of ducks per hectare may range from 100 to 3,000. It is best to release fish fingerlings that are larger than 10 cm while rearing fish with ducks; else, the ducks may eat the fingerlings. The size of the pond and the quantity of ducks released there affect the fingerling stocking density as well. Silver carp, who eat on phytoplankton, as well as catla and common carp, which feed on zooplankton, are the best fish to use in duck-fish culture because nitrogen-rich duck manure increases both phyto and zooplankton production. In duck-fish culture, the fish rearing period is typically maintained at one year, and at a stocking density of 20,000/ha, a fish production of 3,000–4,000 kg/ha/year has been achieved. Additionally, good quantities of eggs and duck meat are also acquired every year.

## 7. Crop livestock fishery biogas/vermicomposting system

- **Agriculture-Dairy- biogas-fisheries farming system.**
- **Horticulture/Agriculture-Goat/sheep-vermicomposting farming system.**

The integration of these businesses can boost overall production while preserving ecological harmony and long-term economic viability. The integrated farming method for small ruminants will also generate income for the farmers, improve soil fertility, enable goats to use weeds as food, and reduce crop disease occurrences. According to Senthilvel et al. (1998), small and marginal farmers in southern Tamil Nadu have seen a significant increase in their income as a result of growing crops+fruit trees+ goats on dry land. Small ruminants can graze feed shrubs and trees directly. Small ruminants can graze feed shrubs and trees directly. This system will thereby reduce labor costs. In this method, small ruminants have grazing periods that last 1-2 weeks and are followed by rest periods that last 3-6 weeks. The recovery time may need to be prolonged in dry conditions. Under this method, small ruminants will be able to move around horticulture plantations, and boundary plantations will supply them with feed during scarcity (Ramana et al., 2011).Horticulture trees will increase the yield for income generating and high quality leaf fodder for small ruminants.

Livestock dung is used to make biogas, which is then used to produce energy, heat, and other things, as well as slurry, which is then used as fertilizer for growing crops. Vermi-compost, which has higher quality as a fertilizer for field crops in terms of high fertility and productivity, can be made from cow dung.

## 8. Silvi-pastoral based farming system with small ruminants

In this method, perennial trees are cultivated on a single plot of land alongside a combination of enhanced pasture species or a variety of grasses. The animals use the tree leaves as feed and for grazing. By addressing the issue of green fodder during the lean season, this technique lowers the cost of concentrate feed for animals. The most common livestock species are sheep and goats.

According to Ramana et al. (2000), during the course of 478 grazing days, lambs and small kids grazing on silvipasture gained weight at a rate of 54.8 and 36.8 g/head/day, respectively, whereas those grazing on natural grasslands recorded weight gains of 41.2 and 26.4 g/head/day. Without any additional concentrate feed, the animal was able to grow weight regularly on both pastures. Due to animal grazing, the fertility of the soil is increased with the addition of vital nutrients from dung and urine. Because of the animals' movements while grazing, leaves and shrubs that are homes to insects and other pests are disturbed; as a result, the frequency of disease will be minimal. Trees provide timber and fodder for animals during lean period.

### 9. Pig-fish based farming system

It has developed a production system for Indian conditions that combines pig farming with fish culture that is both scientifically precise and commercially profitable. Pig dung is either thrown directly into the pond, retrieved from the animal house, and deposited in the pond. Pig stalls are constructed on or near the back of the pond. Pig manure is the finest fertilizer for ponds because it improves the biological activity of the water, which in turn promotes the growth of fish (Devendra and Pezo, 2002).

Additionally, fish consume pig excrement directly, which is a 70% digestible source of food for fish. There is no further need for pond muck or fish feed with this arrangement. Pig emissions, which make up 60% of the cost of fish culture inputs and can replace fish feed and pond manure, have greatly lowered the amount spent on fish culture.

### 10. Rabbit -fish based farming system

The rabbit house is built with embankments in the rabbit-fish integration so that waste and washing may be deposited right into the pond. The pond's 1.0 hectares can be fertilized with the excretions of 300–400 rabbits. By stocking 15000 fingers per hectare per year, it is possible to produce 3500 to 4000 kg of fish.

## Principles of Integrated Livestock Farming System

The Principles of integrated farming systems (ILFS) are to:

1. **Cyclic**
2. **Rational**
3. **Ecologically sustainable**

1. **Cyclic:** The farming system is essentially cyclic (organic resources – livestock – land – crops). Provide a continuous and predictable income and revitalize and improve the productivity of the system. Therefore management decisions related to one component may affect the other.
2. **Rational:** By providing farmers with technology solutions that are both economically and environmentally sustainable and that make wise use

of local resources, crop residue usage may be made more rationally, which helps to reduce poverty.

3. **Ecologically sustainable:** By controlling pests and diseases organically, managing cropping systems, and using less chemicals, the integrated livestock farming system has created agro-ecological balance (pesticides and inorganic fertilizers). As a result, it protects the environment, increases income, and preserves the earth's natural resources.

## Scope of Integrated Livestock Farming System

A variety of resource-saving techniques constitute ILFS, which aims to maximize production levels and profitability while reducing the negative repercussions of intensive farming and protecting the environment. ILFS imposes a great emphasis on good resource management in order to boost farm output, minimize environmental damage, enhance the standard of living for farmers who are limited on resources, and maintain sustainability. A technique known as integrated farming attempts to emulate the natural order by using a variety of plants, animals, fish, birds, and other aquatic flora and fauna throughout the year in addition to crops, livestock, poultry, fish, tree crops, plantation crops, etc. are all examples of farming enterprises.. Particularly for small and marginal farmers, a combination of one or more operations with cropping, when selected, planned, and followed, yields better returns than a single enterprise. To integrate the businesses that will be merged with agricultural producing activity effectively, the farm must be thought of and planned as a unit. Farm enterprise integration will depend on a variety of aspects, including:

1. The area's climate and soil characteristics.
2. The availability of capital, labor, resources, and land.
3. The amount of resource utilization at that moment.
4. A proposed integrated farming system's economics.
5. A farmer's managerial capabilities.

An ILFS can be used to improve a variety of circumstances and conditions in the context of India. The introduction of ILFS is typically carried out in the following circumstances:

- The farmer wants to improve the soil's quality level.
- The farm household often struggles to afford food or lives in extreme poverty.

- Ponds or river-charged overflow zones are employed to store water on farms.
- Fertilizers are expensive or the recommended combination is not easily accessible.
- The usage of inorganic fertilisers has caused an increase in soil salinity.
- The farmer wants to boost revenues from his current holding.
- Water or wind erosion is destroying the farm.
- The farmer wants to use less chemical pesticides.
- The farmer wishes to cut costs associated with waste disposal or pollution.

## Advantages of Integrated Livestock Farming System

ILFS is a multidisciplinary whole farm approach and very effective in solving the problems of small and marginal farmers. The strategy involves merging different farm enterprises and recycling crop residues and byproducts on the farm itself in order to increase income and employment from small holdings.

1. **Productivity:** ILFS offers the chance to boost economic yield per unit area per unit time by intensifying associated livestock-related businesses.
2. **Profitability:** Reduction in manufacturing costs, integration of waste material utilization, and removal of middleman intervention in the majority of inputs used. The fertilizer that can be produced on-site at a farm is free. Farmers' purchasing power is increased as a result of the increasing cost-benefit ratio.
3. **Sustainability:** By utilizing the by-products of linked components effectively, organic supplementation offers the chance to sustain the production base's potential for significantly longer periods of time.
4. **Balanced Nutrition :**A farmer's family can consume a variety of foods, including vegetables and pulses, fruits, eggs, milk, and meat products, to meet all of their nutritional needs.
5. **Environmental safety:** By combining the right components, waste materials are successfully recycled, reducing environmental pollution. Slurry is used as fertilizer and dung as biogas is used in various cooking, lighting, and engine processes.
6. **Recycling:** Effective recycling of waste material (crop leftovers and livestock wastes) using less external inputs (fertilizers, agrochemicals, feeds, energy, etc.).

7. **Income for the year-round:** The interplay of businesses with crops, eggs, milk, mushrooms, honey, cocoons, and silkworms results in a year-round flow of income for farmers. The farming family's labor and land resources have a larger net return.
8. **Energy conservation:** It is facilitated by the use of biogas as a fossil fuel for cooking, electricity, and motor fuel for water pumping.
9. **Resolving the fodder shortage:** It involves planting perennial legume fodder trees along field edges and nitrogen fixation. By-products and crop waste can usefully utilized as fodder, and products like wheat can be fed to chickens and pigs.
10. **Employment generation:** Combining agriculture and livestock enterprises would dramatically boost the labor required and help in greatly decreasing the issues with underemployment. ILFS offer considerable room for hiring seasonal family labor.

## Limitations of Integrated Livestock Farming System

1. Lack of knowledge on sustainable farming practices.
2. Absence of different farming system models.
3. A lack of accessible credit options with affordable interest rates.
4. Absence of some marketing infrastructure, particularly for perishable goods.
5. lack of storage space
6. Lack of education and information in farming communities, especially among young people in rural areas.

## What is arable farming?

Cultivating crops in fields that have typically been tilled before planting is known as arable farming. Arable crops typically need to be replanted every year because they are seasonal. Cultivating crops like wheat and barley on arable land is an alternative to growing fruits and vegetables or raising livestock. It is employed to meet the growing demand for food. It can be done mostly in small-scale, commercial settings or on expansive farming operations.

## Why incorporate livestock in the arable rotation?

Introducing animals to the rotation can have a number of benefits, including enhancing soil health and weed control. The goal is to boost arable fields' productivity, especially those that have been labeled as underperforming. Working with other farming businesses allows for the diversification of income sources and the distribution of production risks, which benefits both sides.

**Opportunities for livestock in the arable rotation of crops for farmers who raise both crops and livestock**

| | Beef and lamb | Dairy | Pigs |
|---|---|---|---|
| Muck-for-staples deals | Yes | Yes | Yes |
| host wintering animals (e.g. dry cows, rearing heifers, beef cattle) | Yes | Yes | - |
| shrinkage in forage crop growth (silage, maize or cover crops) | Yes | Yes | |
| Consented to grazing or cut ( up to one year) | Yes | Yes | |
| Farm Business Tenancy Agreements (such as those for Outdoor Pig) | Yes | Yes | Yes |
| Joint ventures (e.g. share milking agreement) | Yes | Yes | Yes |

Source: (Knight et al., 2019)

# 3

# Drivers and Tradeoffs in Integrated Livestock Farming Systems

*Hina Ashraf Waiz*

## Drivers

- Unique aspects of the local climate and soil.
- Availability of resources and land labor.
- The current level of resource use.
- Economics of the proposed integrated farming.
- Farmer's management skills

Farming systems are one of the main factors determining land use and cover, and their overall effects can significantly alter land surface on a broad scale. These changes are one of the most significant forces behind how human activity affects ecosystem services. Both direct and indirect effects of livestock production on land usage exist. The extensive pasture and grassland utilized for cattle grazing is the source of the direct impacts, while the production of feed is the source of the indirect consequences. Approximately 25% of agricultural land worldwide is used for grazing, and 15% is dedicated to fodder crops (McDemott et al., 2010). Furthermore, the intensification of land use for the production of food and feed has a detrimental effect on biodiversity and other ecosystem services. Grasslands encourage the interdependence of ecosystem services since they can provide agricultural production as well as other ecosystem services. Grassland would also boost cattle productivity without requiring pesticides, which are instead utilized in the production of fodder.

## Tradeoffs in integrated livestock farming systems

Tradeoffs, by which we mean exchanges that happen as compromises, are widespread when land is managed with several goals in mind. Trade-offs is created between agricultural productivity and other ecological services.

Expansion of agricultural land is the primary cause of declines in ecosystem services.

It is essential to analyze the sources of trade-offs and synergies across ecosystem services in order to better understand the connections between livestock production and other ecosystem services and to identify strategies in farming systems to avoid trade-offs through various methods described as under.

### 1. Livestock and sustainable intensification

Although livestock are essential to assure rural areas have access to food, urban demand for animal products is rising quickly. Livestock may be the sole option in dry areas where growing crops is unfeasible, but mixed crop-livestock systems, which are more prevalent in areas with higher rainfall, are essential for maintaining nutrient cycles and traction. Through increased and improved feed availability, enhanced feeding procedures, and genetic advancements, livestock output can be intensified. Additionally, better animal management may have a good impact on agricultural productivity. Crop-focused treatments including the use of inorganic fertilizer, the application of improved seed, conservation agriculture, and small-scale automation can all be made more effective by improving nutrient recycling of manure and more effectively using animal traction.

### 2. Understanding trade-offs between competing goals

The potential trade-offs that could occur for livestock development programs are discussed in the parts that follow. These trade-offs were chosen to encompass environmental, economic, and social factors.

### A) Environmental impact

It is well known that livestock production systems have an adverse influence on the environment. These effects include negative greenhouse gas emissions and land degradation as well as biodiversity loss, effluent positive and ecosystem services. An increase in production efficiency is a key priority for sustainable intensification, with the idea that, via realizing productivity gains in their livestock systems, smallholders' contribution to environmental impacts may be decreased. This assumption is mostly based on modeling at the global and local scales (Smith et al., 2017).

### B) Small holder profit improvements

The main reason that livestock keepers switch to more intensive systems is to increase their revenue or lower their risk, particularly in areas where land or labor are in short supply. In many cases, intensification raises production, and higher output equals higher earnings. Additionally, the livestock business may become more effective, generating more or the same amount of outputs with less inputs, improving household earnings and minimizing harmful environmental effects. For instance, a variety of studies have revealed that smallholder dairy cattle systems with improved animals and effective management exhibit growth in production, more effective input usage, and higher earnings (Dayanandan, 2011; Herrero et al., 2013b).

### C) Gender role

Livestock is a valuable resource for women. In ILFS, women handle many tasks because the male household members frequently work in distant agricultural fields or relocate during lean agricultural seasons. Women are becoming more involved in farming operations as a result of their increased integration into farms, particularly those that generate revenue from home. Most of the time, women are seen working in the following fields: rearing poultry, raising cattle, milch cows, rearing goats and sheep, sewing, growing and selling vegetables, and reforestation in nurseries. Farm women have more access and authority over farm resources. Women do not need to travel far to get resources because many of them are generated on the farm, including fodder and chicken eggs. The women sell several farm products in local marketplaces as well, providing them with some cash income (Kristjanson et al., 2014; Rubin et al., 2010).

### D) Human nutrition and food security

The necessity of ensuring food security for the expanding human population and halting the rapid loss of precious biological diversity stand out as the two biggest problems the world is currently facing. The current global food security scenario is insufficient to ensure food security at various sizes (i.e., on a national, local, or individual basis), and as a result, some or all parts of the world must overcome food insecurity for its vulnerable population (Hoffmann, 2010). ILFS, that are frequently established traditionally, preserve farm output and the availability of a variety of foods year-round so that the entire household is sustainably nourished. ILFS would provide better food diversity than conventional farming. In that sense, ILFS addressed the issue of food security in a holistic manner. Through the availability of animal proteins and vegetables/fruits, ILFS leads to improved household food consumption, especially for the vulnerable family members (children, pregnant/lactating women, and ill). Despite the fact that actual data on food intake in IFS is not frequently available, it has been found to promote food security in numerous scenarios (Takahashi et al., 2016).

### E) Food safety and zoonotic disease

The fundamental relationship between human food consumption and human health must therefore be taken into account in sustainability intensification measures. For example, it has been shown that more and more urban meat markets are selling produce of "poor quality" that has a high prevalence of gastrointestinal sickness (Atherstone et al., 2016). The presence of mycotoxins (such as aflatoxins), which are produced by fungi are found on many major crops used for human consumption and livestock feed, is another illustration of concerns about food safety. Aflatoxins contamination of feedstuffs can affect livestock production and raise additional questions about the safety of human foods derived from contaminated animal sources). If system intensification levels continue to rise, animal numbers and movements increase, urban produce is processed more, and processed feed crops are used more frequently for livestock feeding than natural pastures, the situation of food safety could deteriorate (Grace et al., 2012a).

### F) Cultural acceptance and multi-functional livestock values

Smallholders' livestock often serve purposes other than just providing food, such as generating draught power and manure for crop-livestock mixed systems and adding value to capital assets. Less material values like dowry payments, status symbols, and ethnic identity are also present. Even certain cattle genotypes have cultural preferences. Such perceptions at the household level may represent important trade-offs with maximizing cattle productivity, and corresponding SI measures must take this into account (Ejlertsen et al., 2013.

### G) Risk

Livestock keepers generally have few coping mechanisms and face high degrees of vulnerability. As a result, their main goal is typically to avoid risk, yet in some cases it may be more important to manage risk than to improve productivity. It is anticipated that in the near future, climate change will make cattle owners more vulnerable. Examples of targeted interventions include the index-based livestock insurance, which was created with the goal of reducing climate-related risk and promoting productivity growth with a focus on pastoralists. To remain competitive production systems are likely to increase reliance on inputs, which can have unrecognized negative impacts (Dorward and Chirwa, 2014).

## 3. Using trade-off information for sustainable intensification

### A) Stakeholders perspective

In a "hierarchy" of larger systems (such as farms in communities, communities in regions, regions in nations, and finally a global perspective), agricultural systems can be thought of as sub-systems. There are more stakeholders, objectives, and perspectives at each level. Minimizing environmental damage and preserving food security are likely to be top priorities at the national and international levels; therefore decisions taken at these levels are likely to accord them more weight than other considerations. Risk-averse livestock keepers at this end of the "hierarchy" deal with regionally and temporally complex systems; their aims may vary, be multiplied, or differentiated based on gender, wealth, or other socioeconomic categories(Ahmadi et al., 2015; Garforth, 2015). For instance, smallholders in Kenya's mixed systems identified the provision of food as their top priority for system reforms. However, the availability of manure and milk sales revenue was consistently recognized as well. Demand for both high producing breeds and low yielding, culturally significant zebu cattle further revealed their variety of goals.

### B) Decision making in complex systems

Any development project that wants to be applied, sustainable, or scalable needs to take a systems thinking approach, where various system components and the relationships between them are identified and taken into consideration. More extensive experience with the UN Sustainable Development Goals implementation indicates that systems thinking needs to become a practice rather than an additional development competency (Klapwijk et al., 2014).

### C) Trade-off management

It is important to keep in mind that with the recognition of different Objectives in a production system and indicators linked with it, there may be a way to minimize undesirable trade-offs in some circumstances. It is probably present at many levels of the hierarchical structure and will influence future interpretation and trade-off analyses (Theriault et al., 2017).For instance, studies have shown that certain food safety issues (such aflatoxin contamination) can be addressed both before and after harvest at a reasonable cost, although there may be difficulties in applying the identified strategies in vast informal regions. Women's organizations can present a chance for the successful provision of extension services Women in Senegalese Fulani villages oversee the production of milk; with the assistance of NGOs and development organizations, women have also set up mini-dairies using milk from local herds.

## Sustainability and ecological advantages of integrated livestock farming system

A cost- and environment-conscious integrated livestock farming system with excellent soil, water, crop, and pest management techniques is a must for a sustainable livestock development. Since the system is self-sustaining and less dependent on outside inputs like seeds, fertilizers, etc., it enables self-sustainability. The approach contributes to sustainability by providing the farming family a well-balanced and nutrient-rich diet as well as lowering cultivation costs and raising profit margins on the same plot of land. The energy flow, water cycle, mineral cycle, and ecosystem dynamics are four natural ecological processes that operate on every farm. The ILFS principles are designed to be harmonized with those of sustainable development by balancing food production, profitability, safety, animal welfare, social responsibility, and environmental care (Smith et al., 2017).

## Economic importance of Integrated Livestock Farming System

By increasing the yield per unit area per unit time, a livestock-based integrated farming system enhances the economic viability of small and marginal farmers. Given that there are multiple components in an integrated farming system, evaluating the system's yields and net returns is crucial. As labor requirements often rise and labor is busier throughout the year than in conventional farming, ILFS generates cash for other households. Desired models can be pushed among farmers based on economic returns. Table 1 and 2 illustrate the ILFS models' economic viability by comparing their high net returns to the systems currently in existence in various Indian states.

**Table 1:** Economic viability of ILFS models developed in different states of the India having equal or greater than one hectare

| States | Prevailing system | Net return | Suggested ILFS Model | Net Returns | References |
|---|---|---|---|---|---|
| Kerala | Rice + Fishery | 181725 .58 | Coconut+ Banana + Poultry + Goat + Cow | 1964503 .57 | Sabu et al., 2020 |
| Telangana | Rice-Maize | 1,38,373 | Crop-dairy-hen-sheep-rabbit-quail-manure | 6,09,160 | Goverdhan et al., 2018 |
| Karnataka | Sole crop red gram, paddy and cotton | 43632.69/ha | Crop – Dairy – Vermicomposting | 151414.3 | Rashtrarakshak et al., 2016 |
| Crop – Dairy (2 cows, 1 buffalo) – Goat | 159071.3 | | | | |
| Crop – Dairy – 3 Sheep – 3 Goat | 183221* | | | | |
| Bihar | Cropping alone (Rice-Wheat) | 53000 | Crop-Fish-Goat | 19900.3 | Kumar et al., 2017 |
| Crop-Fish-Cattle | 14000.4 | | | | |
| Crop-Fish-Duck-Goat | 21500.9* | | | | |
| Telangana | | | Paddy-Brinjal-Cotton-Goat | 36918.4 | Srinika et al,. 2017 |
| Paddy-Okra-Cotton-Dairy-Poultry | 49307.8 | | | | |
| Paddy-Tomato-Cotton-Goat-Poultry | 42434.8* | | | | |
| Karnataka | Crop (Maize, cotton, Bengal gram, vegetables) | 58,488/ha | Crop-Dairy-Poultry-Vermicompost -Fishery | 1,50,170/ha | Desai, 2015 |
| Rajasthan | Crops-Dairy (Cow and buffalo) | 33385 /ha | Crop-livestock-horticulture (Fruit, Vegetable and flowers) | 52161 | Singh et al., 2011 |

*System had higher benefit cost ratio

**Table 2:** Economic viability of ILFS models developed in different states of the India having equal or less than one acre.

| States | Prevailing system | Net return | Suggested ILFS Model | Net Returns | References |
|---|---|---|---|---|---|
| Mizoram | Fish only (Rohu, Silver carp and Grass carp) (0.06 acre pond) | 15545.2 | Fish-pig | 48023.19* | Sahoo & Singh, 2015 |
| Fish-poultry | 33664.06 | | | | |
| Punjab | Cropping (Rice + Wheat) | 32,328 per acre | Crop-Dairy-Fish farming | 53,030 | Singh et al., 2020 |
| Nagaland | | | Agriculture-Horticulture-Fishery-Piggery (5 pigs) | 24394 per acre* | Kumar et al., 2018 |
| Agriculture-horticulture-fishery-poultry (50 bird), mushroom unit and Azolla (15 $m^2$) | 32040 per acre | | | | |
| Agriculture-Horticulture-Fishery with a duckery unit at the bank of pond. | 11720 per acre | | | | |
| Horticulture-Fishery-Piggery (3 pigs) | 14840 per acre | | | | |
| Bihar | Rice – Wheat | 46122 /2 acre | Rice-Wheat-Vegetable-Dairy-Fishery | 150865 | Kumar et al., 2012 |
| Telangana | | | Paddy-Brinjal-Cotton-Goat | 36918.4 | Srinika et al,. 2017 |
| Rice-Vegetable-Fruits-Poultry-Goat-Beekeeping | 128693 | | | | |
| Chhattisgarh | Crop + 2 bullocks + 1 cow | 14184 | Crop-2 Bullocks-1 Cow-1buffalo -10 Goats- 10 Poultry -10 Ducks | 33076 | Ramarao et al., 2006 |

# 4

# Integration of Various Components of Farming Systems

*Hina Ashraf Waiz*

## System of Integrated Farming Components

Four main categories can be used to distinguish the components of an integrated farming system.

### (I) Crop husbandry and Horticulture

It is the cultivation and production of edible crops.

**Examples:** Cereals, Pulses, Oilseeds, Spices, Plantation crops, Fodder/forage crop, etc.

Horticulture is the cultivation of fruits, flowers and vegetables and plants for ornament and fancy purposes.

**Examples:** Fruits, Vegetables, Flowers and fancy plants

### (II) Livestock and Poultry

Domesticated animals reared in agricultural settings to produce labor and goods including meat, eggs, milk, fibre, leather, wool, and fur are referred to as livestock.

**Examples:** Cattle, Buffalo, Goat, Sheep, Pig and poultry

### (III) Aquaculture /Fishery

The cultivation of fresh water and salt water fishes under controlled population.

**Examples:** Composite fish, culture, Fingerling production etc.

### (IV) Secondary Agriculture

It includes Bee keeping, cultivation, sericulture, Vermicomposting, Biogas production and Azolla cultivation

## 1. Apiculture/ Bee keeping

It is the common maintenance of bee colonies by humans in hives made of man-made materials. The majority of these bees are honeybees from the genus Apis, however there are others that make honey, like Melipona. There are also stingless bees kept. A beekeeper raises bees to produce bees for sale to other beekeepers or to collect honey and other goods that hives generate, such as beewax, propolis, flower pollen, and bee pollen, to fertilize crops. An apiary, often known as a bee yard, is a place where bees are kept.

## 2. Sericulture

It is the cultivation of silk worms to produce silk.

## 3. Mushroom cultivation

It is a technical process. Early in the Netherlands' tradition of cultivating mushrooms, composed was scooped into the mushroom trays before being injected with spores. Following a nine week delay, flushing could begin, the mycelium hatched sufficiently, and hand harvesting of the grown mushrooms became possible.

## 4. Agro-forestry

It is a system of land use management wherein trees or shrubs are cultivated close to or amid pastureland or agricultural land. There are several advantages to this strategic blending of forests and agriculture, including enhanced biodiversity and reduced erosion.

## 5. Biogas plant

It is a mixture of gases generated when organic matter breaks down in the absence of oxygen. Manure, agricultural waste, plant material, sewage, green waste, and food waste are examples of raw materials that can be used to make biogas. It is a renewable source of energy.

By combining the four aforementioned elements together, an integrated farming system can be developed. (I+II, I+III, II+III, I+IV, II+IV, III+IV, I+II+III, I+II+IV, I+III+IV, II+III+IV, I+II+III+IV).

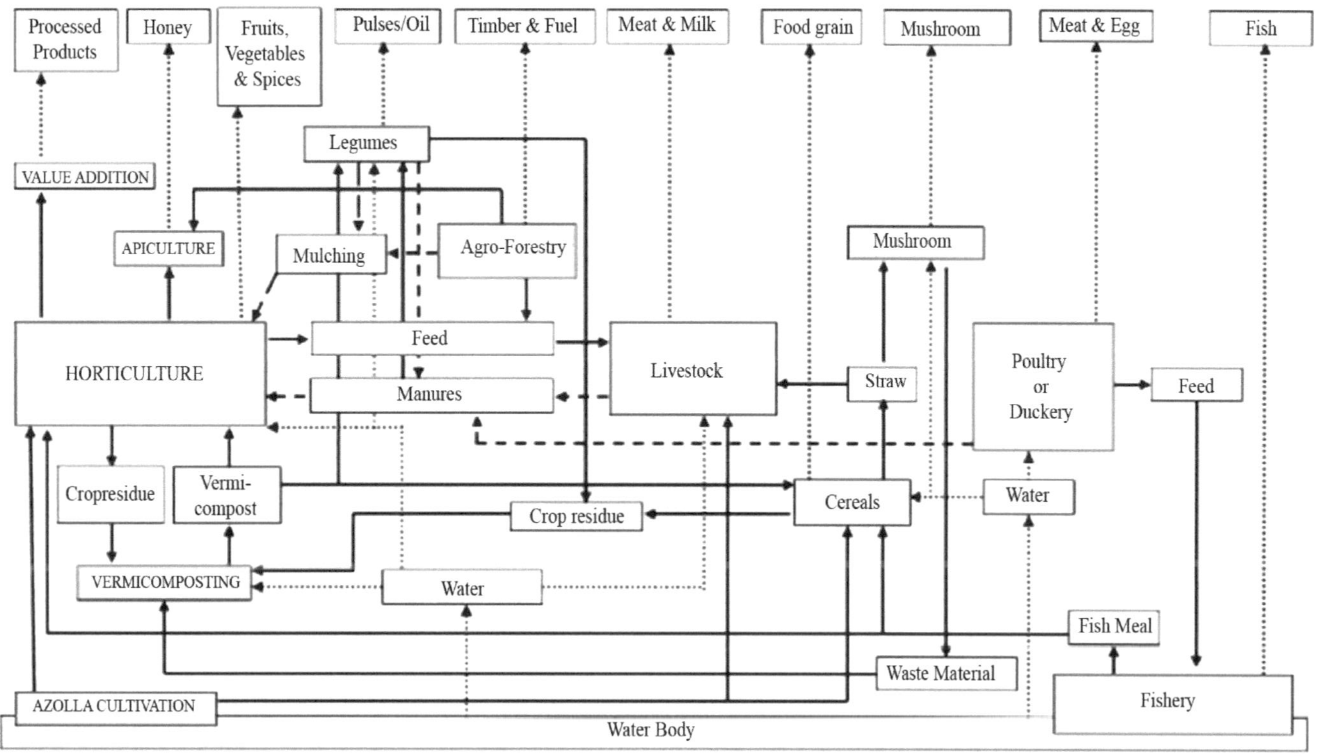


Conceptual framework of integrated farming system, integrating various components of integrated farming system.( *Source* : SS Roy et al. 2014)

## Elements of integrated farming system

1. Watersheds
2. Farm ponds
3. Bio-pesticides
4. Bio-fertilizers
5. Plant products as pesticides
6. Biomass
7. Biogas plant
8. Solar energy
9. Green manuring
10. Vermin-composting
11. Farm yard manure
12. Rain water harvesting

### 1. Watersheds

A watershed is an area of land that feeds all the water running under it and draining off into it a body of water. It combines with other watersheds to form a network of rivers and streams that progressively drain into larger water area.

### 2. Farm ponds

A farm pond is a sizable earthen pit that has been created, typically in a square or rectangular shape. Farmers are capable of carrying perform farming tasks and apply sufficient agricultural inputs.

### 3. Bio-pesticides

Bio-pesticides are certain type of pesticides derived from such natural materials as animals, plants, bacteria and certain minerals. Canola oil and baking soda are two examples of bio-pesticides that have pesticide uses.

### 4. Bio-fertilizers

Bio-fertilizer is a substance which contains living micro-organism, which when applied to seeds, plant surfaces or soil, colonizes the interior of the plant and promotes growth by increasing the supply or availability of nutrients to the host plant. Bio-fertilizer increases yield by up to 30% because of the nitrogen and phosphorous they add to the soil. They also reduce effect of harmful organisms in the soil such as fungi, nematodes.

### 5. Plant products as pesticides

Salt spray, mineral oil, citrus oil, soap-orange citrus oil and water, onion and garlic spray and eucalyptus oil are common plant products used as pesticides.

### 6. Biomass

Organic material derived from living or recently dead organisms is known as biomass, and examples include crop leftovers, animal waste, forested debris, municipal solid trash, etc. Carbon and other molecules including oxygen, nitrogen, and hydrogen make up 75% of the molecules in biomass. A few alkali metals, alkaline earth metals, and heavy metals are also present.

### 1. Biogas plant

#### What is biogas?

The term "**biogas**" refers to a combination of gases produced by the anaerobic breakdown of organic materials, such as food waste, municipal trash, plant residue, and other types of waste. Biogas is made up of methane, carbon dioxide and a small amount of hydrogen sulphide, and moisture.

### Properties of Biogas

The composition of biogas, which is a mixture of several substances, changes according to factors such as the properties of the feed and the degree of degradation. Methane makes up 50 to 70 percent of biogas, along with 30 to 40 percent carbon dioxide and trace amounts of other gases. Combustible gases include methane. The amount of methane in biogas determines how much energy it contains. The range of methane content is between 50% and 70%. The following table 3 and 4 lists the content and characteristics of the biogas.

**Table 3:** Composition of biogas

| Name of the gas | Composition in biogas (%) |
|---|---|
| Methane ($CH_4$) | 50-70 |
| Carbon dioxide ($CO_2$) | 30-40 |
| Hydrogen ($H_2$) | 5-10 |
| Nitrogen ($N_2$) | 1-2 |
| Water vapour ($H_2O$) | 0.3 |
| Hydrogen sulphide ($H_2S$) | Traces |

**Table 4:** Properties of biogas

| Properties | Range |
|---|---|
| Net calorific value ($MJ/m^3$) | 20 |
| Air required for combustion ($m^3/m^3$) | 5.7 |
| Ignition temperature ($^0C$) | 700 |
| Density ($kg/m^3$) | 0.94 |

## Production of biogas

The process is broken down into three stages: hydrolysis, acid generation, and methane production.

### 1. Hydrolysis or Liquidation Stage

The majority of digester feed stocks contain fats, also known as lipids, because they are components of both organic and animal matter. While certain lipids in digester feedstock contain more complex structures, the majority are glycerol and long-chain fatty acid components. There are two types of long-chain fatty acids: saturated and unsaturated. Regardless of the number of chains, extracellular enzymes cause complex long chains of organic molecules to break down into simpler shorter ones. These chemical compounds are broken down by certain enzymes. For instance, one of the enzymes, amylase, hydrolyzes carbohydrates like starch and glycogen into a disaccharide.

### 2. Acid Formation Stage

This second stage involved the conversion of the fermented intermediate materials into acetic acid (CH3 COOH), Hydrogen (H2) and Carbon Dioxide (CO2) by bacteria, which react in acidic medium. The bacteria (acidogenic and acetogenic) use up all the oxygen present creating an anaerobic environment for the methane-producing microorganisms to react afterwards. They also reduce the compounds with a low molecular weight into alcohols, organic acids, amino acids, carbon dioxide, hydrogen, sulphide and traces of methane. Extremely modest changes in the amount of energy required to break down one unit of substrate are indicative of the elimination of oxygen.

### 3. Methane Formation

The final stage of the process is the methane producing stage, which involves methane-producing bacteria called methanogenic bacteria. Methane forming bacteria are sensitive to pH and conditions should be mildly acidic (pH 6.6-7.0) and certainly not below pH 6.2. In the absence of oxygen, these bacteria transform the substances produced during the second stage into substances with a low molecular weight, such as methane and carbon dioxide.. Both acidogenic and acetogenic bacteria and the methanogenic bacteria act in support of one another in that the anaerobic condition created could be poisonous to those bacteria if not used up by other bacteria while the methanogenic bacteria could not also operate without such an environment. The reaction is as shown below:

$$\text{Organic matter} = \frac{\text{Anaerobic}}{\text{Microorganism}} = CH4 + CO2 + H2 + H2S$$

(Price & Cheremisinoff, 1981)

## Biogas plant and its Components

**Mixing tank:** The biogas plant consists of dome like structure. The mixing tank is where the feed material (dung) is gathered. Once enough water has been added, the material is thoroughly combined to create homogeneous slurry.

**Inlet pipe:** The inlet pipe or tank is used to discharge the substrate into the digester. The mixture being digested in the digester tank during anaerobic digestion is referred to as the **substrate.**

**Digester:** The digester is a sealed chamber where the anaerobic decomposition of organic matter takes place. After a few days, the organic matter completely decomposes to generate gases like methane, carbon dioxide, hydrogen and hydrogen sulphide

**Gas holder:** also known as a gas storage dome is where the biogas is collected and stored until it is needed for use.

**Outlet pipe:** Either the outlet pipe or the digester's built-in opening is used to discharge the digested slurry into the outlet tank.

**Gas pipeline:** The gas pipeline transports the gas to the stove or lamp where it will be used

**Raw materials used for biogas production:** Although cattle dung, poultry litter, and agricultural waste can also be used, traditionally, cattle dung has been the primary raw material for biogas plant.

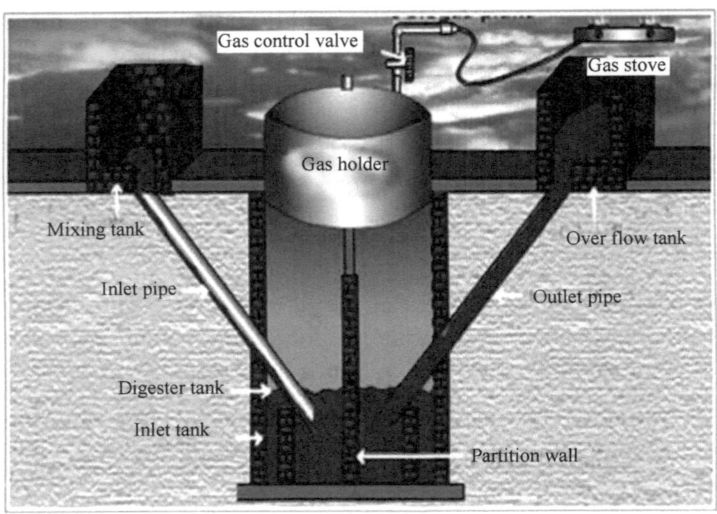


## Classification of biogas plants

Biogas plants may be roughly categorized into three types based on the method of feeding, and they are as follows:

1. **Batch type:** The organic waste materials to be digested under anaerobic condition are charged only once into a reactor-digester. The feeding continues at regular intervals, and after the digestion is finished, the plant is emptied. Typically, retention times range from 30 to 50 days. It only occasionally produces gas. Fibrous materials work nicely with these plants. The two primary drawbacks of this sort of plant are that the digestive process needs to be started with the addition of fermented slurry and that it is expensive to maintain.

2. **Semi continuous:** The digester is charged with a predetermined amount of feed material mixed with water at predetermined intervals of time (once per day), and the digested material (effluent), equivalent to the volume of the feed, flows out of the digester from the other side (outlet).

3. **Continuous type:** The digester is continuously charged with feed material, and the digested material is discharged at the same time (effluent). The primary characteristics of these plants include continuous gas generation, a need for a limited digestive area, a shorter digestion time, less maintenance, etc.

The biogas plants and other biomass are utilized as the feed material for the semi-continuous biogas plants used in the villages to produce biogas. Following is an explanation of semi-continuous type biogas plant categorization.

**A) Floating drum type – KVIC model**

**B) Fixed dome type model – Deenbandhu model**

**A) Floating drum type (Constant pressure)**

In these kinds of plants, the circular digester is formed of bricks. Usually, it is built underground to reduce heat loss from the plant. For larger capacity facilities, partition walls are built (splitting the digester into two portions) to prevent the short-circuiting of digested slurry with the fresh feed. To store the gas created during digestion and serve as an anaerobic seal for the procedure, a separate gasholder is built and installed. As the rate of gas production rises, the level of the drum begins to climb; if the gas is removed from storage, the level of the drum falls. Drum rotation in both the clockwise and anticlockwise directions can help break up scum that has built up in the digester. During gas production, a central guide frame is installed to retain the gasholder and permit vertical movement. Mild steel makes up the drum, which accounts for around 60% of the total plant expenditures. The weight of the drum aids in releasing the gas produced at a steady pressure, and the storage capacity of gas can be determined visually, among other distinguishing characteristics of this type of plant.

Small brick tanks are built to mix cow dung with water and discharge the digester's slurry. To move the raw and digested slurry into and out of the digester, concrete pipelines are available. The top of the drum has a gas outlet pipe to allow gas to escape. The schematic diagram of the KVIC floating drum model, which is primarily used in India, is shown in above diagram.

### Advantages

1. A higher gas production is achieved per unit of digester volume.
2. The rotating action of the floating drum's welded braces helps to break up the sludge.
3. There are no gas leakage issues.
4. Constant pressure of gas..

### Disadvantages

1. It is more expensive since steel and cement are required to construct it.
2. The metal gasholder allows heat to escape.

3. Depending on the humidity of the area, the gasholder required painting once or twice a year.
4. The flexible line that connects the gasholder to the main gas pipe needs to be maintained because the sun's UV rays destroy it.

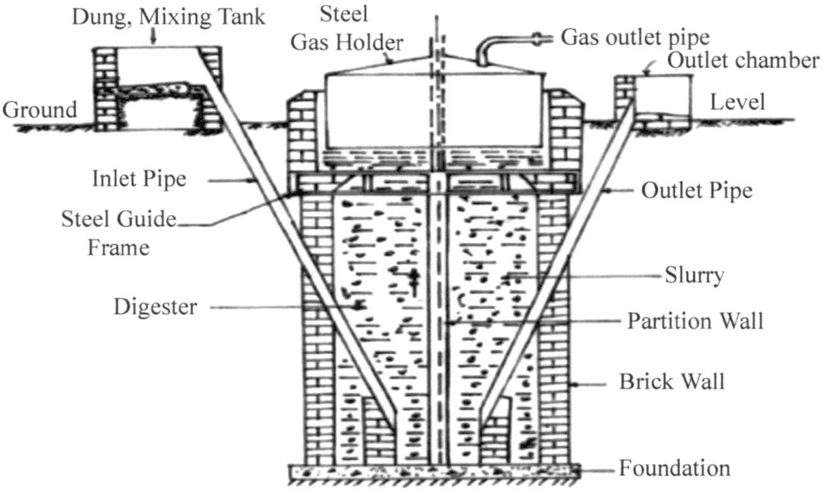


**KVIC model biogas plant**

(Source: Sooch et al. 2013)

## B) Fixed dome biogas plants (Constant volume)

Researchers have developed fixed dome plants that use a dome as a gas container rather than an expensive drum to lower the cost of biogas plants. Designed as a single unit, the gasholder and digester, these plants' digesters are entirely underground in order to preserve the ideal conditions for anaerobic fermentation and prevent dome cracking from temperature and moisture variations.

### Janatha Biogas Plants

It is developed entirely in India. The raw and digested slurry's inlet and outflow are constructed as tanks. In the digester, anaerobic fermentation of the slurry is permitted. As a result, gas is created, which rises and collects in the dome. The slurry is pushed down by the rising gas pressure in the dome, which also raises the slurry level in the intake and outflow tanks. As the gas in the dome is used up, these levels decrease. The pressure required to lift the gas to the consumption point is provided by this displacement. In contrast to floating drum type pressure, which is continuous, the dome's pressure is variable. The total amount of slurry displaced between the inlet and output tanks is equal to the volume of gas stored in the plant.

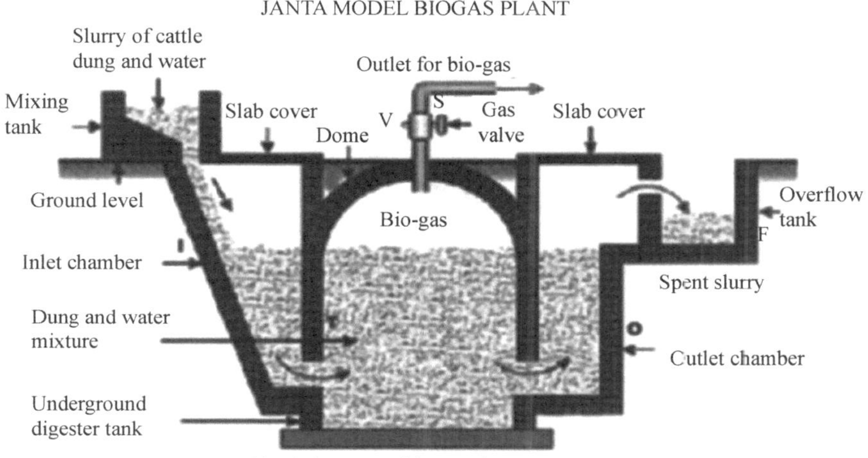


(*Source*: Sooch et al.2013)

## Deenbandhu Biogas Plant

The Deenbandhu biogas plant design is among the best biogas plant designs used in the Indian biogas development program. It is the modified version of Janatha biogas plant model. In 1984, a nonprofit organization called Action for Food Production (AFPRO) in New Delhi created this model. The building was built with materials that were readily available locally, and the business needed skilled laborers to complete the project.

The cost of the bricks used to build the digester wall is decreased by linking the two spheres at their bases, which have differing diameters. The plant's top portion is shaped like a hemisphere, while the bottom portion is constructed as a fragment of a sphere. The digested sludge is removed from the digester through a tank in this facility while feedstock is delivered by concrete pipelines. The outlet hole is built 150 mm lower than the bottom of the gas outlet pipe as a safety measure to prevent the entry of slurry via the pipe. 33% of the plant's total capacity is used for gas storage. According to studies, the Deenbandhu biogas plant costs between 30 and 45 percent less than the Janatha and KVIC biogas plants. The schematic diagram of the deenbandhu biogas plant model is shown in the image below.

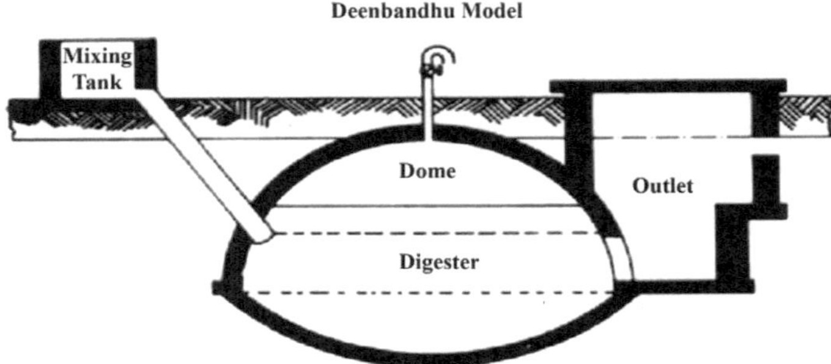


(*Source:* Sooch et al.2013)

## Advantages

1. It is less expensive than the floating drum type since it simply requires cement and no steel. It has non-corrosion trouble.
2. It this type heat insulation is better as construction is beneath the ground.
3. Temperature will be constant.
4. Cattle and human excreta and long fibrous stalks can be fed.
5. No maintenance.

## Disadvantages

1. This type of plant needs the services of skilled masons, who are rather scarce in rural areas.
2. Gas production per cum of the digester volume is also less.
3. Scum formation is a problem as no stirring arrangement
4. It has variable gas pressure

## Factors affecting biogas production

There are many factors that affect biogas production and these factors may have either positive or negative impacts on the biogas production. Biogas digestion is a microbial process, and for that matter requires the maintenance of suitable growth conditions for biogas producing bacteria. The common factors involved in microbiological methanation are:

### 1. Temperature

There are three main temperature mediums for the production of biogas in the digester which are Psychrophilic, Mesophilic and Thermophilic temperatures.

## 2. Nutrients Availability

A sufficient number of nutrients necessary for the growth of the organisms must be present in the waste that will be fed into the digester.

## 3. Retention time (flow-through time)

The retention time is influenced by the composition and the ambient temperature. Batch or continue type facilities are two ways to estimate retention time. While the batch approach provides the most accurate measurement of retention time, the continue type method can only provide an approximate estimate of retention time, as indicated by:

$$\frac{\text{Digester volume}}{\text{Daily feed rate}}$$

## 4. Level of pH

For the methanogenic bacteria to operate normally, a proper pH level is crucial. The methanogenic bacteria like a pH of 7 to 7.2. (Ghosh & Klaus, 1978). Between 6.5 and 7.5 is the optimal pH range for methane production. Normal pH values for animal waste fall within this range (Moulik, 1990).

## 5. Nitrogen inhibition and C/N ratio

Microorganisms require carbon and nitrogen as fundamental building blocks for their metabolic processes. The ideal C/N ratio ranges from 8 to 20, depending on the specific situation, and is necessary for the methanogenic bacteria to function at their best. Other elements that may affect the formation of biogas include inhibitory ones like the detergent in sewage sludge, heavy metals, moisture content, and cations.

### Advantages of Biogas

1. **Non-polluting**: As there is no smoke produced during the burning of biogas, no hazardous gases, such as CO2, CO, NO2, or SO2, are released.
2. **Reduces the Need for Landfills:** Slurry leftover from the production of biogas is used as manure on farms. There is no need for landfills because the method of disposal is reliable and safe.
3. **More affordable technology:** Biogas plants can be installed for very little money and become self-sufficient in 3 to 4 months.

4. **Generate employment:** Many people are given job chances, especially in rural areas.
5. **Renewable source of energy:** Because the production is reliant on waste generation, an unending process, it is seen as a renewable source of energy.

## Disadvantages of Biogas

1. **Not effective enough on a large scale:** It is not feasible economically to utilize biogas on a large scale since it is difficult to increase its efficiency.
2. **Contains impurities:** It has several contaminants that are challenging to manage even after several purifying cycles. When biogas is compressed to be used as fuel, the container is severely corroded.
3. **Unstable and possibly hazardous:** Methane interacts violently with oxygen to form carbon dioxide. Methane is highly flammable, which makes it prone to explosions.

## Uses of biogas

The energy requirements of modern society can be met by biogas as a suitable alternative fuel. It can be used to generate electricity, cook, light, and other things. Figure illustrates the flow.

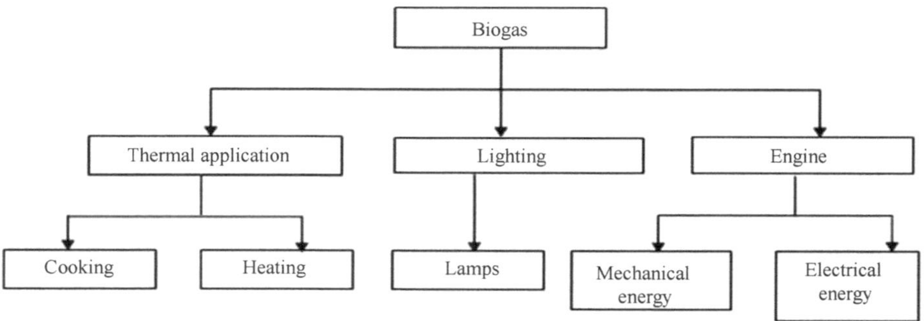


## 1. Cooking and lighting

Biogas is primarily used in homes for cooking and lighting. Stoves that can burn biogas effectively must be properly made since biogas differs from other regularly used gases, such as propane and butane, in terms of its qualities and is only accessible at low pressures (4 to 8 cm of water). A key advantage over conventional cooking fuels like firewood and cow dung cake is that biogas burns with a blue flame and produces no soot or odor.

An electric generator or a gas mantle can be used to provide lighting. Biogas mantle lamps provide a lighting capacity equal to 40 W incandescent bulbs at 220 volts and consume 2-3 ft3 per hour. The majority of these areas are rural and without electricity.

## 2. Biogas as an Engine Fuel

In both fixed and mobile engines, biogas can be utilized as fuel to supply motive power, pump water, power machinery (such as threshers and grinders), or even produce electricity. Both spark ignition engines and four-stroke diesels can be run on it. Biogas energy production is a tested and commercially viable technique. Typical installations make use of biogas-compatible spark-ignited propane engines. Other on-farm uses for biogas-fueled engines are also a possibility. Small internal combustion engines and generators can be utilized to generate power in rural areas with densely populated areas, supporting decentralized forms of electricity and preventing grid losses.

## 3. Use of biogas as vehicular fuel

Without further processing, biogas is useful as a fuel for the majority of purposes. However, the presence of CO2 is unacceptable if it is to be utilized to power cars for a variety of reasons. It reduces the engine's power output, takes up space in the storage cylinders (cutting down on the vehicle's range), and can result in problems with freezing at valves and metering points where the compressed gas expands during operation, refueling, as well as during the compression and storage procedure. Therefore, in addition to compressing the gas into high-pressure cylinders that are carried by the vehicle, the raw biogas must be cleaned of all or the majority of the CO2 to make it suitable for use as a vehicle fuel.

## 4. Uses of bio digested slurry

After digestion, the digester's slurry, which is rich in various plant nutrients like nitrogen, phosphorus, and potash, will be rinsed out. The physical, chemical, and biological qualities of the soil are improved by well-fermented biogas slurry, which increases both the quality and quantity of food crop yield. The biogas plant's slurry is more than just a soil conditioner; it improves soil texture and supplies and releases plant nutrients. It is highly advised for use in farming because the slurry no longer contains parasites and pathogens. If slurry is used effectively, according to its economic value, an investment can be recovered in three to four years.

Following digestion inside the digester, the cow dung slurry has the following attributes and advantages:

- Effluent is odorless when fully digested and does not draw flies or other insects when left out in the open.
- Termites are attracted to raw dung and can harm plants treated with farmyard manure (FYM), whereas effluent repels termites and reduces weed growth by around 50%. It has a higher fertilizing value than FYM or fresh dung and promotes more rapid weed growth when FYM is employed.
- Crops can readily absorb nitrogen in the form that is readily available.

### 8. Solar energy

It is powered by solar energy. This energy can be used to produce electricity, heat the water in our homes, etc.

### 9. Green manuring

It is the process of lowering into the earth beneath composed green plant tissue. The green manure's function is to enrich the soil with organic matter.

### 10. Vermi-composting

In the vermicomposting process, earthworms turn organic waste into manure with a high nutritious content. They are frequently observed residing in soil, consuming biomass, and excreting it in a digested state.

Worm cultivation is known as "**vermin-culture**." Earthworms consume organic waste and release "**vermin-casts,**" which are excreta that are high in nitrates and minerals including phosphorus, magnesium, calcium, and potassium. These are applied as fertilizer to improve the soil's quality.

### Vermicomposting comprises two methods

1. **Bed Method:** This is a simple technique for creating beds of organic stuff.
2. **Pit Method:** Using this technique, organic waste is gathered in pits made of cement. However, because to issues with inadequate aeration and waterlogging, this method is not widely used.

## Vermicomposting procedure

The following describes the full vermicomposting process:

### Aim

The production of vermin-compost using earthworms and other biodegradable waste.

### Principle

The major purpose of this procedure is to enrich the soil with nutrients. A natural fertilizer called compost facilitates the smooth passage of water to developing plants. Since they consume the organic materials and make castings as a result of their digestive processes, earthworms are mostly used in this procedure.

The following nutrients constitute the vermin-compost nutrient profile: 1.6% Nitrogen, 0.7% Phosphorus, 0.8% Potassium, and 0.5% Calcium,0.2% magnesium 175 ppm of iron, 96.5 ppm of manganese, and 24.5 ppm of zinc are present.

### Materials Required

Water is a necessary component.

- Cow dung.
- A thatched roof.
- Sand or soil.
- Gunny sacks
- Earthworms.
- Herbal biomass
- A sizable bin (plastic or cemented tank).
- Leaves and dry straw collected from paddy fields.
- Biodegradable trash gathered from fields and kitchen.

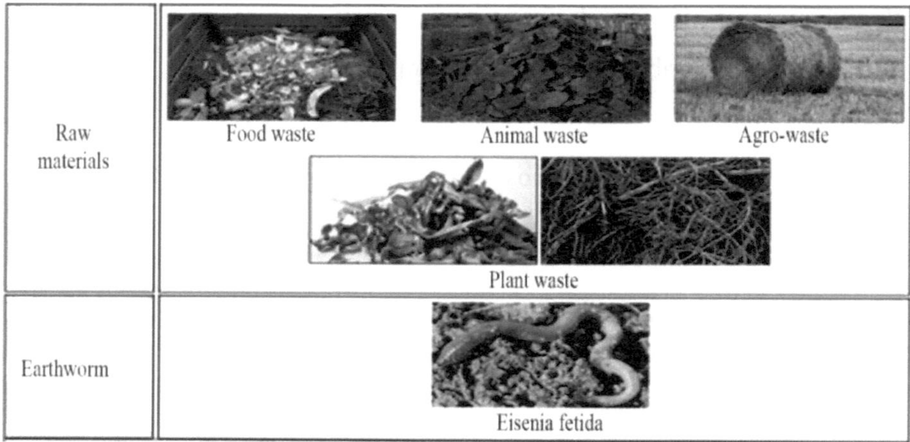


## Procedure

1. A concrete or plastic tank can be used to prepare compost. The tank's size is determined by the availability of raw materials.
2. Collect the biomass and expose it to the sun for approximately 8 to 12 days. Use the cutter to cut it to the desired size now.
3. To hasten decomposition, prepare cow dung slurry and scatter it over the mound.
4. Fill the tank's bottom with a layer of soil or sand that is 2 to 3 inches thick.
5. Use decomposed cow manure, dried leaves, and other biodegradable scraps obtained from the fields and kitchen to make fine bedding. Distribute them evenly over the sand layer. Continue layering the tank with the chopped bio-waste and partially digested cow dung until it reaches a depth of 0.5-1.0 feet. Continue layering the tank with the chopped bio-waste and partially digested cow manure until it reaches a depth of 0.5-1.0 feet.
6. After incorporating all of the bio-waste, scatter the various earthworm species over the compost mixture and cover it with gunny bags or dry straw.
7. Water the compost frequently to keep it at the proper moisture level.
8. To keep out ants, lizards, mice, snakes, and other pests and to shield the compost from rains and direct sunlight, cover the tank with a thatch roof.
9. Keep an eye on the compost frequently to prevent overheating. Keep the temperature and humidity appropriate.

## Results

The raw materials are all transformed into vermi-compost after the 24th day, when 4,000 to 5,000 additional worms are added.

## Advantages of using vermin-compost

The principal advantages of vermicomposting are:

1. Helps plants develop their roots.
2. Enhances the soil's physical structure.
3. By using vermin-compost, the soil becomes more fertile and water-resistant.
4. Promotes plant growth, germination, and agricultural yield.
5. Provides plant growth hormones, such as auxins, gibberellic acid, etc., to the soil.

## Disadvantages of Vermicomposting

Vermicomposting has the following severe disadvantages:

1. The process of transforming biological stuff into forms that can be used can take up to six months.
2. It emits an extremely repulsive smell.
3. Vermicomposting needs a lot of attention. Regular feed addition is required, and it's important to take precautions to prevent over feeding the worms.
4. Neither a dry bin nor a wet bin should be utilized. It is vital to regularly monitor the moisture levels.
5. They promote the development of infections and pests including fruit flies, centipedes, and flies.
6. Vermicomposting produces black, nutrient-rich soil from kitchen garbage and other green waste. It keeps the soil in good health because of the microorganisms that are there.
7. Vermicomposting is an environmentally friendly method for turning organic waste into compost and producing beneficial nutrients.

## Farm yard manure

Farmyard manure (FYM) is a decomposed mixture of residual roughages and feed that have been supplied to the animals, as well as faeces, urine, litter, and other animal waste products. A well-decomposed FYM contains 0.5-1.5% N, 0.2-0.4% P2O5, and 0.5-1.0% $K_2O$. FYM, a good source of organic carbon, activates the biotic life of the soil's flora and fauna. Farmyard manure is utilized as a natural fertilizer and helps the soil's structure. It boosts the soil's ability to store more nutrients and water. In order to improve the soil's mineral supply and plant nutrients, it also boosts its microbial activity.

## Preparation of Farmyard Manure

- To prevent it from being too moist and being exposed to direct sunlight, collect the cow dung and urine into an even layer beneath a straightforward roof. More dung, urine, and water are added if the mixture becomes too dry.
- Farmyard manure can be used to fields as fertilizer in roughly six months.
- Three to four weeks before to planting crops, manure spreaders can be used to add partially digested farmyard manure to the soil.
- The manure will breakdown more quickly and deliver nutrients to the soil thanks to this exposure to the elements.
- The nutrients in the soil may be washed off by heavy rain if a significant time passes between spreading the manure and growing the crops.
- If the manure has aged long enough, it can be applied right before planting the crops. Vegetable and fruit crops benefit from the use of farmyard manure.

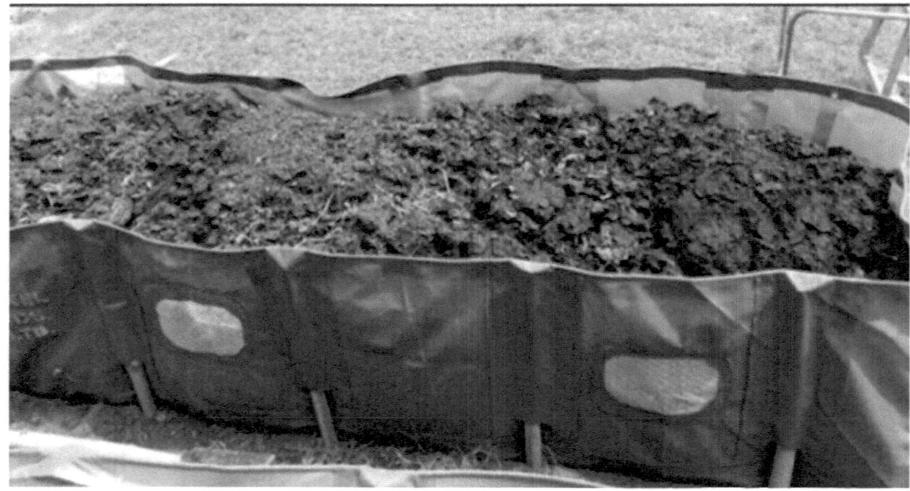

Source: Sahu et al. 2020

## Processing of farm yard manure

The cattle shed's daily collections of dung and urine-soaked waste are placed in trenches that measure 6-7m in length, 1.5–2 m in width, and 1m in depth. Each trench is filled up to a height of around 0.5 m above the ground. Cow dung earth slurry plaster needs to be applied to the heap's top, which should be fashioned like a dome. It's ready to apply after three to four months. For each cow, this technique may prepare 7 to 8.5 $m^3$ of manure annually.

## Factors affecting nutritional built-up of FYM

1. **Age of Animal:** Growing animals and milk-producing cows keep the nitrogen and phosphorus necessary for productive processes like development and milk production in their systems, and the excreta do not contain all of the plant food elements present in the meal. Inferior older animals excrete more waste, including waste from their body tissues, than they do consume.
2. **Feed:** When the feed has a lot of plant food components, the amount of excreta produced is also improved.
3. **Nature of litter used:** Leguminous plant debris and cereal straw were both used as litter, which increases the nitrogen content of the manure.
4. **Manure ageing:** As manure ages, it gets richer and less bulky.

## Advantages of FYM

- Organic material and slowly-released nutrients from farmyard manure enhance the soil and help it retain water and nutrients.
- It helps to break down heavy soils. Farmyard manure adds texture to sandy and light soils.
- Farmyard manure is an organic, easily accessible supply of nitrogen.
- Worms are attracted to the soil and make excellent mulch when farmyard manure is applied.

## Disadvantages of FYM

- Some micronutrient availability is decreased.
- Its disintegration pollutes the atmosphere by releasing toxic chemicals into it.

- When compared to fertilizer, handling, storing, and applying FYM requires a higher cost per unit weight of nutrients..

## 12. Rainwater harvest

It is the collection and storage of rainwater for on-site reuse as opposed to letting it runoff. The gathered water is guided to a deep pit reservoir via percolation (a well, shaft, or borehole).

## Types of Integrated Farming Systems based on several enterprises

- Crop-livestock-fish farming system (CLFFS)
- Crop-livestock-poultry-fish farming system (CLPFFS)
- Crop-poultry-fish-mushroom farming system(CPFMFS)
- Crop-fish – poultry farming system(CFPFS)
- Crop-livestock-fish-vermicomposting farming system (CLFVFS)
- Crop-livestock-forestry farming system(CLFFS)
- Agri-silvi-horticulture system (ASHS)

The above mentioned integration models have been discussed in the previous chapter in detail.

## Integrated farming system types based on the agro-ecosystem

Integrated farming systems can be broadly classified into four categories depending on the ecosystem:

1. Irrigated low and uplands.
2. Rainfed and dryland areas.
3. Hill regions.
4. Island

### (i) Irrigated upland integrated farming system

A variety of crops and types can be cultivated owing to the controlled irrigation system. Irrigated uplands provide a wider range of component alternatives than lowlands and rain-fed lands. It is simple to incorporate the elements of an irrigated upland farm, **including dairy, poultry, goats, sheep, pigs, mushrooms, apiaries, pigeons, and rabbits**. Along the edges of the fields and the farm, multipurpose farm forestry trees can be grown in addition to perennial trees like coconuts and other fodder trees.

**Examples of Irrigated Upland integrated farming system**

- Crop + Dairy + Biogas unit.
- Crop + Poultry + Biogas unit.
- Crop + Sheep / Goat rearing + Biogas unit.
- Crop + Sericulture.
- Crop + Piggery.

### (ii) Irrigated Lowland integrated farming system

The primary crop in the lowland is rice. An integrated farming system can include fish, chicken, duck, and mushrooms in the lowlands. It is thought to be less dangerous to cultivate food in low land because of the availability of available water (wetlands). Lowland soils are often rich in nutrients and have a heavy texture.

**Examples of Irrigated lowland integrated farming system**

- Rice + Fish + Azolla
- Rice + Fish + Poultry
- Rice + Fish + Poultry –Mushroom
- Crop + Pigeon + Goat
- Crop + Piggery + Duck

### (iii) Rain-fed and Dry-land integrated farming system

The dry-land ecosystem has low crop yields, limited crop variety, poor and marginal soils, inadequate and inconsistent rainfall distribution, and low value crops. Due of the limited crop season (4-5 months), people are unemployed for the rest of the year. Dry-land farmers can improve their standard of life and increase their employment options by diversifying their cropping by incorporating elements like livestock (sheep/goat husbandry), silvi-culture, horticulture tree crops, and pastures.

**Examples of rain-fed and dry-land integrated farming system**

- Crop + Goat
- Crop + Goat + Agro forestry
- Crop + Goat + Agro forestry +Horticulture

- Crop + Goat + Agro forestry +Horticulture + Farm Pond
- Crop + Goat + Buffalo + Agro forestry + Farm Pond

### (iv) Hilly Regions integrated farming system

This method is typically used in hilly, high-altitude areas where it is impossible to construct terraces or irrigation systems across slopes. This strategy combines soil and water conservation with forestry, agriculture, cattle, and fisheries. From protected hilltop slopes, rainwater is collected in a pond with seepage control. Before runoff water enters the pond, sediment retention tanks are built at a number of locations. The pond's water level determines everything regarding the cultivation.

### Examples of hilly regions integrated farming system

- Agriculture + Horticulture
- Agriculture + Horticulture + Livestock
- Agriculture + Horticulture + Fisheries +Livestock
- Agriculture + Horticulture + Silvi-culture
- Agriculture + Horticulture + Livestock
- Agriculture + Livestock

### (v) Island integrated farming system

Models of integrated farming systems have been developed for the Andaman and Nicobar Islands

### Examples of island integrated farming system

- Coconut + cum + fodder + cum + milch cattle
- Coconut + cum fish culture in salt affected lands
- Fruits + fodder + milch cattle
- Cocunut + cum + fodder + cum + fish or prawn culture

# 5

# Solar and Wind Energy Utilization

*Hina Ashraf Waiz*

It is believed that efforts to combat poverty and advance sustainable development must include both the development of livestock and energy-related activities The relationship between energy and livestock in alleviating poverty is less clear and has just recently grown increasingly significant, despite the fact that each of these issues has been identified separately(Steinfeld et al., 2006). The livestock industry has an effect on many different environmental resources and requires careful maintenance because land, soil, water, and biodiversity are becoming increasingly scarce. The interaction between livestock and renewable energy sources may be beneficial to both sectors.

## Renewable energy

Any energy that derives from essentially infinite natural resources is referred to as renewable energy (such as water, sun, wind, and animal or plant biomass). This is either because these resources have enormous energy reserves or because they have the ability to naturally regenerate.

It does not harm the environment and is not exhausted because it comes from natural resources, some of which, like the sun, are abundant or are resources that can be found anywhere in the world. As a result of the ongoing search for affordable and environmentally responsible solutions across a variety of industries, renewable energy has gained increased recognition on a global scale

## Characteristics of renewable energy

1. **Inexhaustible:** Due to the fact that it is produced using natural, completely renewable resources that are unbounded, its supply may be sustained across time
2. **Pollution free**: As the word "renewable energy" implies, it is a clean energy source that does not generate waste that pollutes the environment, and as a result, it does not cause pollution.

3. **Competitive**: After the initial investment is required to assure its successful operation, the costs are generally low, making it a competitive energy. It is an energy source that may be used for many different purposes, but its main advantage is that it encourages long-term economic growth.

## Advantages of renewable energy for farms

- It never runs out because it comes from renewable natural resources and may be used forever, reducing dependency on conventional energy sources.
- As a result, it is seen as a viable option for all future energy needs of humanity.
- It doesn't emit any greenhouse emissions.

## Types of renewable energy

### 1. Solar energy

Sunlight is the source of solar energy. There are two types:

A) **Solar Photovoltaic**: This technology absorbs solar energy and turns it into electricity using photovoltaic panels.

B) **Solar Thermoelectric**: it is also called a solar thermos; heat is produced using solar energy, which may be used to cook food and warm water. The energy of the sun is controlled by use of mirrors or lenses.

C) Different levels of solar energy utilization exist. On a small scale, it is used in homes for lighting, cooking, water heaters, and solar-powered homes; on a medium scale, it is used for irrigation and water heating. Solar power is used locally for rural electrification, water pumping and purification, and vaccine refrigeration.

## Solar-powered refrigerators and freezers

- Health clinics typically use solar-powered refrigerators and freezers because of their high dependability, low maintenance requirements, and the importance of a reliable preservation technique for vaccinations.
- Off-grid freezers that use propane or kerosene are still less expensive than photovoltaic (PV) refrigerators in terms of cost. It is a serious problem since most electric refrigerators require a lot of energy and

were not designed to be powered by PV systems.

- PV systems become less competitive as a result of the requirement for bigger refrigerators that use a lot of energy to prepare dairy, fish, and meat. On the other hand, hybrid PV/diesel and PV/wind systems have been used to power larger refrigeration systems in places like Mexico and Indonesia.
- The freezing of vaccines for veterinary use is another application for PV refrigeration in the agriculture industry, where dependability and minimal maintenance needs are crucial considerations. One example of this type of application is the project on rangeland management in the Syrian Steppes, which is handled by the FAO.

## Solar-powered irrigation for livestock

As livestock operations expand, more watering holes and natural water sources are needed. Effective watering systems are also needed to improve the supply of high-quality water and to safeguard watercourses.

- Using PV pumps to hydrate livestock is one of the alternatives that are growing in popularity in off-grid areas.
- PV systems don't need monitoring or a fuel source, are portable, and require less maintenance. Solar-powered pumping systems typically do not require a battery for energy storage because energy is typically stored in the form of water in a water reservoir, which lowers maintenance costs and improves system dependability.
- PV system investment costs are still significant, which limits their appeal to large herds.
- Developed markets can be found in countries like Australia, Brazil, Mexico, the United States, and Western Europe. There are many commercially available PV pumps for animal irrigation. The Mexico Renewable Energy Program has been advocating the use of PV pumps for cow hydration in Mexico as one of the most enticing PV uses.

## Advantages

The benefit of the system for the livestock industry in nations like Mexico is that the system's several large-scale cattle owners manage their herds over a huge region, necessitating a number of modest pumping systems to enable constant rotation of their cattle. On existing lands, greater milk and meat production as well as better natural resource management are the key immediate effects.

### Disadvantages

Unrestricted access to a body of water has negative potential effects that could be life-threatening, such as:

- Impact on the watercourse, damaging the vegetation and water banks;
- Faecal pollution, introducing pathogens and excessive nutrients into the water leads to negative effects on the health of the herd, such as decreased water consumption, leg and hoof damage, and a rise in water-transmittable infections.

### 2. Wind power

It is the energy produced by using wind energy.The electrical generators-connected mills are propelled by the wind. Poor livestock keepers who have trouble accessing water sources may find it advantageous to use wind energy to pump water for their animals. Utility-scale turbines can produce anywhere

### 3. Hydroelectric power

It is the power that the river currents use to generate their energy.

### 4. Marine power

It is the energy that the waves of the ocean carry.

### 5. Biomass and biogas

Utilizing organic material is how this kind of energy is produced. It is created by igniting organic animal or plant waste.

### 6. Geothermal energy

It is the energy that the Earth generates and holds in reserve. It has the capacity to produce both heat and power. It is always found in deposits below the surface of the earth, usually in volcanic areas.

### Solar energy in the poultry

Some entrepreneurs have begun to use photovoltaic solar energy for poultry production farms in the poultry sector. This sector uses the most of this type of renewable energy. Additionally, it helps prevent system fluctuations, which frequently lead to losses in bird production.. This reduces electricity consumption while also preventing system oscillations. For a poultry farm, electricity is both the most expensive and most necessary running expense. A flock of chickens can perish in seven minutes if the fans and tunnel ventilation system in the housing aren't powered during the hot seasons. Another benefit of using this energy is that it increases the process's energy security because it lessens its reliance on fossil fuels, among other things. The carbon footprint is also diminished.

## Solar-powered lights for poultry

Artificial illumination lengthens the day, encourages chicken growth, and increases egg output. Another essential component for reducing the mortality rate of chicks on poultry farms in particular regions is heat. In conventional chicken farms, **"heat lights"** are utilized to provide both heat and light. In hot regions, ventilation is required, and electric fans driven by solar panels are the best option.

# 6

# Newer Approach for Changing Farming Systems in the Light of Global Warming

*Lokesh Gautam*

## Effects of climate change on livestock, including mitigating and adaptation measures

The number of people is expected to increase from 7.2 billion to 9.6 billion by 2050. (UN, 2013). This represents a 33% increase in population, but the demand for agricultural products will climb by approximately 70% during the same time period as the global quality of living rises (FAO, 2009). Livestock is essential for ensuring food security. Meat, milk, and eggs make up 34% of the protein consumed globally; they also contain essential micronutrients such vitamin B12, A, iron, zinc, calcium, and riboflavin. Because they supply 33% of the world's protein consumption and 17% of its calorie consumption, livestock products are a crucial agricultural product for ensuring the safety of the world's food supply.

The rapid increase in demand for livestock products in developing nations is referred to as the "livestock revolution." In a changing climate, hundreds of millions of vulnerable people depend on livestock because it can adapt to hard conditions and endure climate shocks. There are several factors that are anticipated to have a detrimental effect on livestock output, including climate change, competition for land and water resources, and food security at a time when it is most needed.

Greenhouse gas (GHG) emissions, which warm the atmosphere, are the principal cause of global climate change (IPCC, 2013). The livestock industry, which produces 14.5% of the world's greenhouse gas emissions, may contribute to increased land degradation, air and water pollution, and a decline in biodiversity, according to Gerber et al. (2013). (Bellarby et al., 2013). Although it is anticipated that demand for livestock products will increase by 100% by the middle of the twenty-first century, climate change will have an impact on livestock production through competition for natural resources, quantity and quality of feeds, livestock illnesses, heat stress, and biodiversity loss (Garnett, 2009). Thus, it might be difficult to maintain a balance between productivity, domestic food security, and environmental conservation.

The following factors determine how the livestock industry will impact global warming and how climate change will affect food security and livestock production.

## Effects of climate change on livestock

Changes in the production and quality of feed crops and forage, animal growth and milk production, illnesses, reproduction, and biodiversity are just a few of the potential effects on livestock. The main causes of these effects are an increase in temperature, an increase in atmospheric carbon dioxide (CO2) concentration, changes in precipitation, and a combination of these factors. Fig. 1 shows the effects of climate change on many facets of animal productivity. Temperature has an impact on the majority of significant factors that affect the production of livestock, such as the availability of water, animal production, reproduction, and health. The quantity and quality of fodder are impacted by changes in CO2, temperature, and precipitation. The main influences of changing precipitation patterns and rising temperatures on livestock diseases.

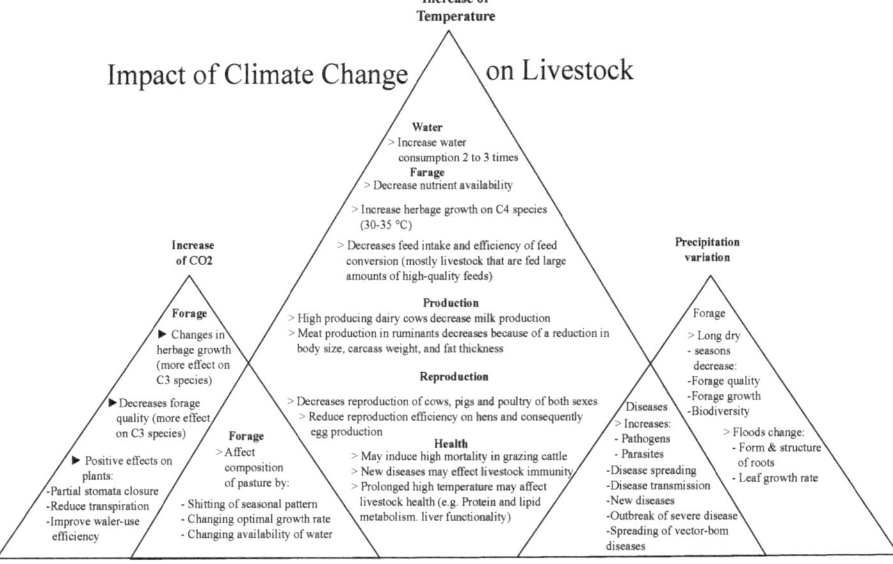


**Fig. 1:** Effects of climate change on livestock (Rojas et al. 2017)

## A. Quality and quantity of feed

- An increase in temperature and atmospheric CO2 levels will be the key factors affecting the quantity and quality of feed.
- An increase in CO2 concentration will alter the growth of herbage, with a greater influence on C3 species and a lesser impact on grain yields (Chapman et al., 2012) The effects of CO2 will be favorable since they lead to partial stomatal closure, reduced transpiration, and enhanced water use efficiency in some plants (Thornton et al., 2015).
- C4 species, which thrive in hotter climates and use water more effectively than C3 plants, make up less than 1% of all plants on Earth. The impacts on C4 species will be larger and could promote herbage growth if the temperature climbs to 30 to 35 C. However, depending on the environment, production technique used, and plant species; the results may vary (Herrero, 2010).
- As a result of variations in optimal growth rates, changes in temperature and CO2 levels will modify the dynamics of species competition, which will alter the make-up of pastures Primary productivity may rise if temperature, precipitation, concurrent nitrogen deposition, and species composition in pastures alter (Polley et al., 2013).
- The quality of feed crops and pasture may be impacted by rising temperatures and dry conditions due to variations in nitrogen and water-soluble carbohydrate content. Temperature rises may cause plants to produce more lignin and other cell wall constituents, which impair plant digestion and breakdown rates and lessen the nutrients available to cattle. However, when the CO2 concentration increases, C3 plants will see bigger gains in the quality of their feed than C4 plants. Furthermore, compared to C4 plants, C3 plants have higher crude protein and are more easily digested.
- Floods and other extreme weather events can alter the form and structure of roots; impair leaf growth, and lower total productivity.
- The quantity and quality of fodder are affected by topography and the length of the growing season. A 2°C increase will have a negative effect on pasture and livestock productivity in arid and semi-arid areas while having a favorable influence in humid temperate areas. The length of the growing season is also an important factor in determining the quality and quantity of fodder because it impacts the length and timing of the forage's availability. If pasture quality deteriorates, methane emissions

per unit of gross energy use can increase. If forage quality deteriorates, it can be required to reduce forage consumption and switch it out for grain in order to prevent animals' increased methane emissions (Polley et al., 2013).

### B. Water

As per Thornton et al., (2009), 70% of all water resources are used by agriculture, making it the largest consumer of fresh water in the world. Although worldwide water consumption is rising, water stress may affect 64% of the world's population by 2025 as a result of water scarcity and depletion. Water supply difficulties will have an impact on the livestock business, which depends on water for animal drinking, feed crops, and product processes..

The amount of water consumed by animals, which makes up around 8% of all human water consumption worldwide, may increase by a factor of two to three as temperatures rise. Crops and cattle must be raised in areas with abundant water supplies or in livestock systems that use less water in order to address this issue (Nardone et al., 2010).

Salination increases the quantities of heavy metal, chemical, and biological toxins already found in water bodies around the world, which could affect the productivity of cattle. Water salinization may affect animal metabolism, reproductive, and digestion. The neurological, skeletal, cardiovascular, excretory, and respiratory systems, as well as the hygienic standard of manufacturing, are all susceptible to damage from heavy metals and chemical contaminants.

### C. Livestock diseases

Climate change may affect livestock diseases, depending on the region, kind of land use, disease characteristics, and animal susceptibility (Thornton et al., 2009). Animal health may be impacted directly or indirectly by climate change, especially increased temperatures. The risk of sickness and mortality is raised as a direct result of the rise in temperature. The indirect effects of climate change are thought to include the ramifications for microbial populations (pathogens or parasites), the expansion of vector- and food-borne diseases, host resistance, and the scarcity of feed and water.

Climate change may alter how diseases spread, lead to major disease outbreaks, or even result in the introduction of new diseases that could harm livestock that isn't usually exposed to them. In order to keep their resistance, livestock must be investigated for disease dynamics and adaptation.

Pests that are spread by vectors like flies, ticks, and mosquitoes are affected by changes in precipitation and global warming. For instance, White et al. (2003) found that increased tick infestations caused animals to lose about 18% of their weight when they estimated the impacts of climate change on Australian livestock. As new diseases develop, there's a fair probability that they will act as a kind of genetic mixing bowl for humans and other animals, permitting the blending of new genetic material and facilitating its transmissibility.

### D. Heat stress

The degree of stress experienced by livestock during severe weather depends on a variety of factors, including temperature, humidity, species, genetic potential, age group, and nutritional state. Livestock at higher latitudes will be more affected by the rise in temperatures than livestock in lower latitudes since cattle in lower latitudes are normally better adapted to high temperatures and droughts (Thornton et al., 2009). Production strategies for confined animals that have better control over climatic exposure will be less affected by climate change. Heat stress has a detrimental effect on forage intake, milk production, feed conversion efficiency, and performance. Hot, humid weather causes heat stress, which affects livestock's behavior, metabolism, and even results in mortality. Use of feed nutrients, feed consumption, animal productivity, reproduction, health, and mortality are just a few results of heat stress in livestock.

### E. Biodiversity

A specific environment's diversity of genes, species, and ecosystems is referred to as that environment's biodiversity, according to Swingland (2001). Populations with little genetic diversity are vulnerable, and one of the main reasons for this biodiversity loss is climate change (UNEP, 2012). 15% to 37% of all species worldwide could become extinct as a result of climate change (Thomas et al., 2004). Increases in temperature have an effect on the distribution, demise, migration, and reproduction of species. The Intergovernmental Panel on Climate Change's Fifth Assessment Report states that a temperature increase of 2 to 3 degrees Celsius beyond pre-industrial levels may result in a 20 to 30% loss in plant and animal species (IPCC, 2014). In 2000, 16% of animal breeds were known. Cattle, goats, pigs, sheep, water buffalo, cattle, and horses were all lost.

Additionally, according to the FAO (2007), of the 7,616 livestock breeds reported, 20% were in danger of extinction and nearly one breed was wiped out every month. The most extinct breeds of all the species taken into account are cattle (N = 209). Chicken (33% of breeds), pigs (18% of breeds), and cattle

(16% of breeds) were the livestock species with the highest percentages of risk of breed elimination. Between 7% and 10% of mammalian species—not just livestock—were deemed to be in danger in developing regions, whereas between 60% and 70% are deemed to be at unknown risk. However, in developed nations with highly specialized and a small number-based livestock industries, the percentage of mammalian species under risk ranged from 20% to 28%.

Animals and plants will be significantly impacted by climate change and the loss of biodiversity. It is critical to conduct additional research into the inherent genetic capabilities of different breeds and discover those that are better able to adapt to changing climatic conditions because some breeds and species cannot be naturally replaced.

### F. Agro-ecological zones

Production and farming of livestock are two examples of agricultural activities that vary around the world. Agro-ecological zones (AEZs) were developed by the International Institute for Applied Systems Analysis and the Food and Agriculture Organization of the United Nations to explain these variations (FAO, 2017). These zones are established based on the climate, landform, soils, land cover, and land use. The five main categories of AEZs are arctic, tropical, subtropics, temperate, and boreal (FAO, 1996). Climate change effects inside an AEZ can generally be good or detrimental. For example, higher temperatures will directly affect the output of livestock by changing the animals' migration and reproductive cycles. Therefore, livestock species with limited habitat, small populations, limited mobility, and low breeding rates will be the most vulnerable.

The majority of ruminants on Earth are found in tropical and subtropical AEZs, notably in dry or semi-arid areas where climatic conditions limit animal productivity and yield. A common climatic factor because of the high temperature is heat stress. For instance, in the tropics and subtropics AEZs of Europe, North America, Africa, and Australia, heat stress increases livestock disease and mortality (Herrero et al., 2012; Renaudeau et al., 2012).

### G. Food security

In many different ways, livestock is essential for guaranteeing food security. The majority of animal feed is unsuited for human consumption; it is produced in regions where it is difficult to grow crops; it is a major source of calories, proteins, and vital micronutrients; and it provides manure for crop cultivation. However, there are concerns that growing animals may jeopardize food security. First, grains are used as feed in the production of livestock, which is a global concern because they are farmed for animal feed and not for human use. As an illustration, in 2002, a third of the global cereal crop was fed to animals. The majority of the feed for cattle is made up of grass and legume forage that grows in places unsuitable for agriculture (O'Mara, 2012), and in many countries, livestock do not receive supplementary grain feed. The presence of livestock in these areas improves the security of the food supply.

Because of a rise in temperature, climate change may cause a reduction in the amount of food that can be digested. Therefore, decreased animal feed intake as well as decreased forage quality and quantity may have an effect on livestock productivity. Because animals use the nutrients that are available to them first for sustaining their physiological demands, then for development or the production of milk, and last for reproduction, these two factors have an impact on livestock output (Hatfield et al., 2008). Due to possible increases in infections and diseases in their diet and effects on the animals themselves, climate change affects the nutritional content of livestock products (Karl et al., 2009).

The efficient conversion of natural resources into human food is necessary to maintain a neutral food balance. The security of the food supply is significantly influenced by animal husbandry. This is made possible by effectively manufacturing protein from cattle (FAO, 2013). Contrarily, this conversion will be impacted by the effects of climate change because they will reduce animal productivity and decrease the nutritious content of products made from cattle.

## 2. Impact of livestock on climate change

Livestock contribute 14.5% of the total annual anthropogenic GHG emissions globally (Gerber et al., 2013). Animal production, feed production, raising livestock, manure, processing, and transportation are all ways that livestock affect the climate (Fig. 2). Manure and feed production release CO2, N2O, and CH4 into the atmosphere, which has an impact on climate change. CH4 emissions increase as a result of animal production. Land use changes and the processing and transportation of animal products both contribute to an increase in CO2 emissions.

According to numerous studies (Reynolds *et al.*, 2010) the cattle production is frequently linked to detrimental environmental effects such as land degradation, air and water pollution, and biodiversity destruction. Increasing livestock production is expected to result from a depleting natural resource base, which will exacerbate environmental damage if natural resource management is not implemented.

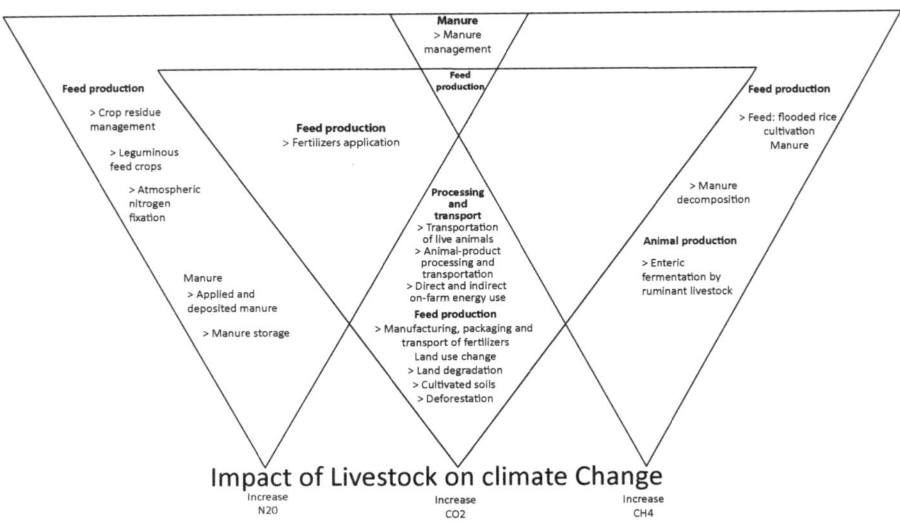


**Fig. 2:** Impact of livestock on climate change on (Rojas et al. 2017)

## A) GHG emissions

The three main GHGs that animals emit are CO2, CH4, and N2O. CH4 is responsible for the majority (44%) of anthropogenic GHG emissions, followed by N2O (29%) and CO2 (27%).Livestock is responsible for 5% of the world's anthropogenic CO2 emissions, 53% of the anthropogenic N2O emissions, and 44% of the anthropogenic CH4 emissions (Fig. 3).

The lower productivity and efficiency of the livestock system as a result of excessive nutrition, energy, and organic matter loss can be linked to higher levels of these gases. Livestock production produces more greenhouse gas emissions than the total global transportation sector. Through a number of factors, including animal physiology, housing for animals, manure storage, manure treatment, land application, and chemical fertilizers, the livestock business contributes to greenhouse gas emissions both directly and indirectly (Casey et al., 2006). Three instances of direct animal emissions are enteric fermentation, respiration, and excretions. The cultivation of feed crops, manure application, farm activities, the processing of animal products, transportation, and the allotment of land for livestock production are among the sources of indirect emissions, according to IPCC (1997). Some of the classical examples are desertification, carbon released from farmed soils, and deforestation.

In the livestock industry, indirect emissions contribute more than direct emissions to the atmospheric release of carbon (Steinfeld et al., 2006).

Using a worldwide livestock environmental assessment model, Gerber et al. (2013) calculated the livestock sector's contribution to anthropogenic GHG emissions, which totaled 14.5% of all emissions (GLEAM). GLEAM analyses the emissions of global livestock production via supply chains. The primary elements of the livestock supply chains that GLEAM examines include herd, feed, manure, animals' energy requirements, feed intake, production, and emissions, allocation of the total emissions at the farm gate (physical farm boundaries) to co-products and services (emission per kg of product), and post-farm gate emissions (transport and processing).

Another type of land use change that GLEAM considers is the conversion of forest to pasture or arable land for agriculture. The sources of the 14.5% of livestock GHG emissions are shown in Fig. 4.Followed by feed production, which accounts for 21.1% of the sector's emissions, land use change, which accounts for 9.2% of emissions, post-farm gate, which accounts for 2.9% of emissions, and direct and indirect energy, which accounts for 1.8% of emissions, enteric fermentation accounts for 39.1% of the sector's emissions (Gerber et al., 2013).Direct and indirect energy, which accounts for 1.8% of emissions.GHG emissions are affected differently depending on the geography and type of farming system, though. For instance, strengthening any of the three main livestock production systems and expanding industrialized (or landless) systems will increase CO2 emissions since these systems use more fossil fuels and less solar energy for photosynthesis (Steinfeld et al., 2006). Gerber et al. (2013) calculated livestock GHG emissions by region and found that Asia generates the highest, followed by Latin America and the Caribbean.

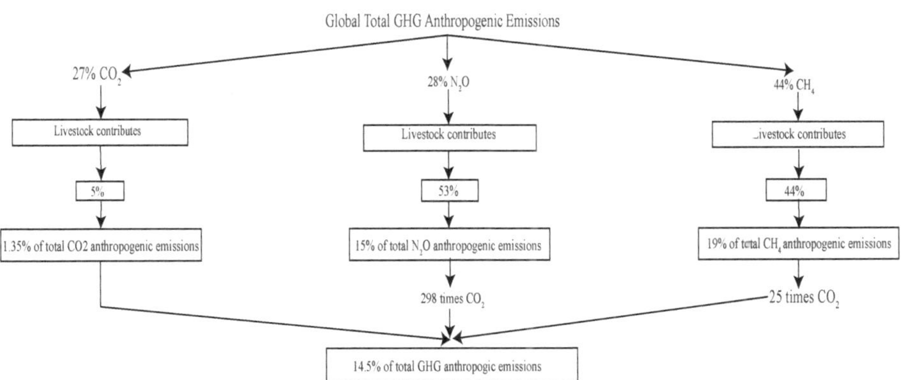


**Fig. 3:** Contribution of livestock to anthropogenic emissions of total greenhouse gases (Rojas et al. 2017).

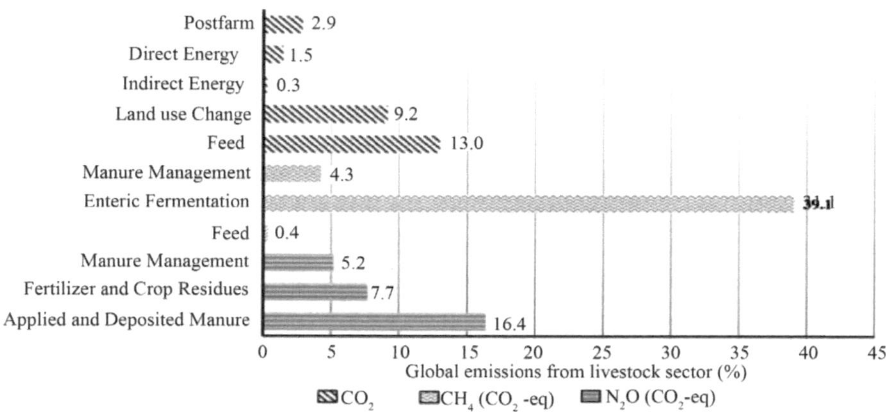


**Fig. 4:** Global livestock sector emissions of greenhouse gases (Gerber et al. 2013) )

## B) Land use

A total of 38.5% of the world's land area is used for agriculture, of which 28.4% is arable land and 68.4% is permanent meadows and pasture (DSI MSU, 2015). Changes in the use of agricultural land are correlated with profit per acre and opportunity cost (Steinfeld et al., 2006). Profit per unit of land is the term used to describe farmers' desire to control a specific land usage. The amount of profit will differ depending on a number of factors, such as the biophysical characteristics and cost of the land, as well as access to markets, resources, and services. The opportunity cost concept calculates the expenses, both monetary and social, of multiple uses of a specific piece of land. Opportunity costs include the costs of private production and ecosystems. Therefore, land use decisions are determined based on private profit per unit of land when there are no related costs for non-marketable ecosystem services.

The natural landscape has undergone tremendous modification as a result of the rising demand for animal products. The phrase "land degradation" is used to describe how the physical, chemical, and biological properties of soil are deteriorating. Due to farmers' exhaustion of their soil resources and subsequent search for more suitable land, one of the causes influencing land to transition from forest to croplands and pastures has been emphasized as land degradation. The natural carbon cycle is impacted by changes in land use, which raises GHG emissions and releases enormous amounts of carbon into the atmosphere. Natural settings, especially forests, store more carbon in their soil and plants than do pastures and croplands. Up to 40% of anthropogenic CO2 emissions are captured by the earth's soil and terrestrial vegetation (The Royal Society, 2001).

The main causes of CO2 emissions include deforestation, cultivated soils, and land degradation brought on by animal grazing. 9.2% of all livestock GHG emissions are attributable to land use change, of which 6% are attributable to the expansion of pastures and 3.2% to the expansion of feed crops. As pasture areas serve as net suppliers of CH4 when soil compaction from cattle hooves limits gas diffusion, the conversion of forest area to pastureland may also diminish the amount of CH4 that soil microorganisms may be able to metabolize. Approximately 28 million tons of CO2 are produced each year by livestock-related cultivated soils, and 100 million tonnes are produced each year by livestock-related pasture desertification, according to Steinfeld et al. (2006).

### C) Feed production

The production of forage and feed crops, feed processing, and feed transportation—all of which include the use of manure and synthetic fertilizers—are the main sources of GHG emissions in the livestock business (IFAD, 2010). These emit 45% of all CO2, N2O, and NH4 emissions from cattle that are caused by humans globally. Due to the production of nitrogenous fertilizers required to grow crops for animal feed, the livestock industry has a considerable impact on greenhouse gas emissions. Natural gas, coal, and oil are all used in the production of fertilizer. When packaging, shipping, and use in the livestock industry are all taken into account, the yearly carbon dioxide emissions from the production of fertilizer exceed 40 million tons. Artificial fertilizers supply 40% of the nitrogen that crops need. Ammonia volatilization loss from synthetic nitrogen fertilizers is a secondary source of greenhouse gas emissions. 4 to 5 million tons of mineral fertilizer is used in the production of animal feed. An average of 14% of the nitrogen in mineral fertilizer is lost due to ammonia volatilization. Therefore, it is anticipated that the cattle business will produce 3.1 million tons of worldwide ammonia volatilization annually from mineral fertilizers (Steinfeld et al., 2006).

$N_2O$ is a different source of GHG emissions. The usage of fertilizers, agricultural nitrogen fixation, and atmospheric nitrogen deposition all tend to enhance N2O emissions. Mineral fertilizer emits 0.2 million tons of N2O-N annually into the atmosphere from the livestock industry. Animal feed crops with high lectin content also contribute to increased $N_2O$ emissions. Steinfeld et al. (2006) increased the area of soybeans used as livestock feed to determine the contribution of alfalfa and clover since there are no estimates of their global production. Leguminous feed crops consequently produce more than 0.5 million tons of $N_2O$ emissions per year. When both contributors (mineral fertilizer and leguminous feed crops) are taken into account, total annual

N2O emissions are 0.7 million tons. As the usage of fertilizer and manure rises, a 35–60% increase in $N_2O$ emissions (0.9–1.1 million tons of total $N_2O$ emissions annually) is projected by 2030. (Bruinsma, 2003).

Nitrogen fertilizer production for feed generates CO2 emissions that are 50% lower than those from the farming of cattle. The cattle industry uses fossil fuels on-farm for a range of tasks, including running equipment, irrigation, heating, cooling, and ventilation systems, as well as making insecticides and herbicides. The production of feed accounts for more than half of the utilization of fossil fuels. On-farm fossil fuel consumption is thought to be responsible for 90 million tons of CO2 annually, with emissions from the rearing of cattle and the manufacturing of nitrogen fertilizers being equal in size.

Since livestock respiration is a part of the global biological system cycle, it is not considered to be a net source of CO2 emissions. The plant that the animal eats is produced when atmospheric CO2 is converted into organic compounds or biomass. The amount of CO2 that is absorbed in a vegetative state is considered to be equal to the amount that animals release. The animal, on the other hand, acts as a carbon sink because some of the carbon it consumes is absorbed in its live tissue and byproducts, such as milk (UNFCCC, 1998).

Livestock's normal digestive processes (enteric fermentation) and manure management account for 44% of the world's anthropogenic CH4 emissions. 80 percent of the 52 different forms of agricultural emissions come from enteric fermentation and manure. Enteric fermentation changes the absorbed feed into digestible feed throughout the animals' digestive process. Through the breath, enteric fermentation releases the byproduct CH4, this by-product is therefore seen as an energy waste. Enteric fermentation and ensuing methane emissions may vary depending on food content and feed consumption. Methane emissions from an animal can be decreased by feeding them more concentrates (Beauchemin et al., 2009).

Different regional factors (such as terrain and temperature) and manufacturing processes have an impact on methane emissions (Gerber et al., 2013). Due to enteric fermentation, ruminant animals (such as cattle, sheep, and goats) release between 87 and 94 Tg of methane per year (IPCC, 2013). Methane emissions from enteric fermentation are produced by grazing systems in 35% of cases, mixed crop-livestock systems in 64% of cases, and industrial sources in 1% of cases. The large percentage of mixed crop-cattle systems means that these systems account for two-thirds of total livestock production. India, China, Brazil, and the United States are the countries with the highest livestock-related methane emissions (IPCC, 2013). India, which has the largest livestock population in the world, produced 11.8 Tg of CH4 emissions in 2003, with enteric fermentation accounting for 91% of those emissions and manure management for 9%. If the linear relationship between methane emissions and animal population holds true, global methane emissions from livestock production might increase by 60% by 2030 (Chhabra et al., 2013).

### 1. Emissions by species and products.

As per Gerber et al., (2013), beef and dairy cattle are the main producers of these emissions; accounting for 65% of all livestock GHG emissions. The remaining 7–10% is made up of small ruminants, poultry, buffalo, and pigs. Beef cow emissions make about 41% of the sector's overall GHG emissions when calculated using commodities. With 20% of the market, dairy cattle come in second, ahead of swine which contributes 9% followed by buffalo (8%), poultry (8%), and small ruminants (6%).

### 2. Enteric fermentation

Enteric fermentation, the primary source of GHG emissions from cattle, buffalo, and small ruminants, is responsible for between 43% and 63% of the emissions from the livestock sector (Fig. 5). However, the production of feed—which also involves the use of machinery, the creation of fertilizer, and the transportation of feed—results in the majority of emissions for hens and pigs (between 25% and 27%). Pigs' enteric fermentation is significantly lower than that of ruminants because their digestive tract produces less methane as a byproduct than ruminants.

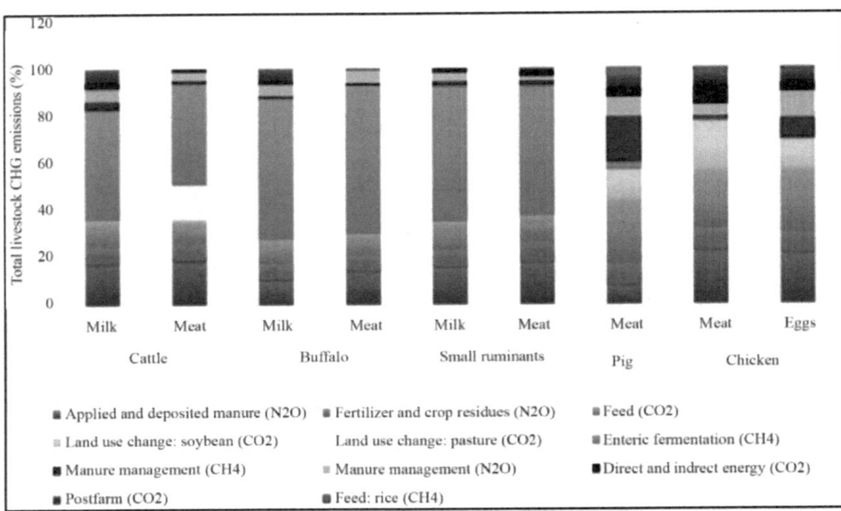


**Fig. 5:** Global GHG emissions by species and commodities (Gerber et al. 2013)

## F) Manure

Excreta from livestock release $N_2O$ and CH4 gas. Methane is produced when the organic components of manure break down in anaerobic conditions. Methane emissions from liquid manure in lagoons or holding tanks are higher. Air temperature, moisture content, pH, storage period, and animal diet are just a few of the variables that affect how much methane is released from manure. The decomposition of manure generates 17.5 million tons of CH4 in annual global methane emissions. About half of all manure-related worldwide methane emissions come from pig dung. China is the nation with the highest global methane manure emissions, mostly from pig dung.

The environment, the disposal procedure, and the handling techniques all have an impact on the $N_2O$ emissions from manure storage. In dry waste-handling systems, it is more likely that manure will initially be handled aerobically, which will release $N_2O$ emissions, and then anaerobically.

The largest source of $N_2O$ emissions worldwide is the application of manure to the land. The soil's organic carbon content, pH, soil temperature, precipitation, and soil temperature all have an impact on how rapidly applied or deposited manure's nitrogen is absorbed by plants or crops. According to Steinfeld et al., 1.7 million tons of manure soil emits $N_2O$ each year (2006). The excreted manure emissions deposited on pasture systems are 40% lower than the applied manure emissions in crop-livestock systems. Systems of mixed agricultural and livestock production emit 90% less $N_2O$ into the environment than do industrial ones.

## G) Processing and transportation

The production of livestock worldwide from "market-oriented intensive systems" and the energy costs of processing animals and their products can be used to estimate global processing emissions (WEC, 2015). The type of livestock system and its size have an impact on how much energy is utilized. More than half of the energy used in confinement systems is used to produce feed, which involves employing technology, seeds, insecticides, and herbicides. Energy is also used extensively by the ventilation, heating, and air-conditioning systems. The transportation of animal products to retailers and feed to livestock farms has an impact on GHG emissions. The largest contributor to GHG emissions in this category is long-distance shipping. The annual $CO_2$ emissions from the transportation of beef were estimated to be between 800-850 thousand tons of $CO_2$ based on FAO statistics for 2001-2003.

## Adaptation and mitigation strategies

Crop and livestock productivity can be increased against the effects of climate change by implementing adaptation measures (USDA, 2013). The effect of cattle on climate change may be significantly minimized with mitigation measures If they are included into national and regional policy, adaptation and mitigation can have a significant influence (Dickie et al., 2014).

### 1. Adaptation measures

Breeding strategies, institutional and legislative changes, scientific and technological advances, a change in farmers' perceptions, and their capacity for adaptation are all examples of adaptation techniques (USDA, 2013). Research on evaluations is needed in order to apply these adaptation techniques and tailor them based on geography and livestock systems. This might be accomplished using global and local scale remote sensing technology.

### 2. Methods for raising and managing livestock.

Diversification of livestock species and crops, integration of livestock systems with forestry and crop production, and changes to the time and locations of farm operations are a few examples of adaptations that call for modifying production and management systems (IFAD, 2010). Farmers can increase their livestock's tolerance for climate-related problems like drought and heat waves by diversifying their crop and animal populations. Additionally, the variety of livestock and crops helps to prevent pest and disease outbreaks brought on by climate change.

Agroforestry is a type of land management that combines agricultural productivity, environmental protection, and carbon sequestration to lower sector emissions. Agroforestry involves growing trees alongside crops and pastures in a mixture. While enhancing biodiversity, air, soil, and water quality, managing pests and diseases, and nutrient cycling, agroforestry may enhance yields.

One sort of adaptation that might increase food security is changes to mixed crop-livestock systems. More than half of the milk, meat, and crops including cereal, rice, and sorghum are produced by this sort of agricultural system, which is already in use in two-thirds of the world. By producing more food on less space with fewer resources, such as water, changes to mixed crop-livestock systems can increase efficiency.

As a measure of adaptation, bettering feeding practices may indirectly raise the efficiency of cow production. Some of the recommended feeding practices include including agroforestry species in the animal's diet and training producers in the production and storage of feed for diverse agro-ecological zones (IFAD, 2010). These methods can, in turn, minimize the risk from climate change by promoting greater intake or making up for inadequate feed consumption, limiting excessive heat load, lowering feed insecurity during dry seasons, and reducing animal malnutrition and mortality (IFAD, 2010). Moving livestock and crop production may reduce soil erosion and improve moisture and nutrient retention.

### 3. Breeding strategies

Animals can improve their breeding practices to increase their resistance to diseases and the effects of heat stress while also promoting growth and reproduction. Furthermore, it will be essential to enact legislative changes that enhance adaptive capacity by making it easier to apply adaptation techniques. Creating an international gene bank, for instance, might enhance breeding operations and act as a global policy.

### 4. Farmers perception and adaptive capacity

One of the obstacles to the success of these changes is the farmers' mindset, which makes it difficult for them to understand the problem and undertake mitigation and adaptation measures for climate change.Therefore, it is important to research how farmers view mitigation and adaptation measures. Open-ended survey questions or group discussions at workshops have been used to investigate individual and group opinions for studies on mitigation and adaptation. Qualitative research is the process of acquiring data on farmers' perceptions. Understanding farmers' viewpoints and including them in the creation of rural policy increases the possibility of attaining goals for food security and environmental conservation.

Education, family farm succession, and social links between farmers and farming communities can all help farmers perceive risk more clearly when making decisions. Barnes (2013) used the latent class clustering method, which produces results using statistical methodology, to assess the variety of risk perceptions among dairy producers on climate change. They discovered that, as a result of climate change, succession planning and family relationships had an effect on risk perception. They suggested increasing the social capital of farming communities to promote acceptance of Communication plans for dealing with climate change and putting adaptation measures into effect.

## Mitigation measures

There are numerous technologies and techniques that can be used to reduce the GHG emissions produced by the livestock industry. However, their utilization is uncommon. Carbon sequestration, improved diets to lessen enteric fermentation, and improved waste management are the best technological solutions for combating climate change. (Fig 6).

## 1. What is carbon sequestration?

Carbon sequestration is the process of diverting carbon dioxide (CO2) from sources of emission and storing it in the ocean, terrestrial environments (vegetation, soils, and sediments), and geologic formations. It may occur naturally or on purpose. Carbon sequestration can be accomplished by reduced rates of deforestation, reversing deforestation by replanting, concentrating on higher-yielding crops with better varieties adapted to climate change, and improving land and water management. A study on the beef sector by Gerber et al. (2013) in Brazil showed that boosting animal and herd efficiency might reduce GHG emissions from grazing land use and land use change by up to 25%. Conservation tillage, erosion control, soil acidity management, double-cropping, crop rotations, enhanced crop residues, mulching, and other practices can all help restore soil organic carbon in cultivated soils.

Through the planting of trees, the improvement of plant species, the inter-seeding of legumes, the introduction of earthworms, and the fertilizing of pastures, better pasture management can also result in the storage of carbon. Additionally, grass production and soil carbon sequestration could be improved by increasing grazing pressure in grasslands with fewer grazing animals than the livestock carrying capacity. Improved grazing land management could globally sequester 0.15 giga tons of CO2-equivalent years.

## 2. Enteric fermentation

Boosting dietary fat content, providing higher-quality forage, increasing protein content, providing supplements (such as feed antibiotics), and using anti-methanogens (vaccines to decrease methane emissions) are a few examples of strategies for preventing enteric fermentation.

A 1% increase in dietary fat can cut enteric methane emissions by 4-5%. To prevent a decline in cow performance, rumens must keep fat content at or below 8% of dry matter. Higher quality feed improves digestibility while simultaneously reducing methane emissions. Increasing the protein level of feed can also make it more digestible while reducing methane emissions overall per unit of product (Martin et al. 2010).

Enteric fermentation can be reduced by introducing supplements like feed antibiotics, which tend to enhance weight gain and lower feed intake per metric ton of meat produced. Cow somatotropin, a bovine growth hormone, encourages milk production. Fewer animals must be utilized in order to produce the same amount of milk, which reduces emissions. Another method that directly reduces rumen methane emissions is anti-methogen vaccination. However, due to the fact that this innovative technology is so recent, it is unknown how successfully it reduces emissions and how it affects animal health.

## Manure management

The majority of methane emissions from manure management are caused by the anaerobic treatment and storage of manure. Despite the potential for nitrous oxide emissions from manure applied to pasture, mitigation strategies are frequently challenging to put into practice because of the manure dispersion on pasture. As a result, the majority of mitigation strategies involve shortening the time manure is held, enhancing when it is applied, utilizing anaerobic digesters, covering the storage, using a solids separator, and changing the diets of the animals.

Anaerobic digestion can lower methane emissions while generating biogas. Manure is stored in lagoons or tanks used as anaerobic digesters where biogas is collected and burned for energy production or flared. This process turns methane into CO2, lowering the possibility of GHG emissions. The greatest way to promote the use of anaerobic digesters is through rules that provide substantial incentives for flexibility. Anaerobic digesters are expensive for producers. By trapping and eliminating methane, covering ponds, tanks, or lagoons can minimize emissions in a manner similar to digesters.

GHG emissions can be decreased by using different storage and handling techniques. Reducing storage duration, enhancing housing and waste management systems to handle manure, and separating bedding from manure using a solids separator are some of these approaches. In confinement systems, the solids separator is primarily utilized to filter out solids from manure streams as they enter the storage or treatment facilities. Methane emissions are decreased, the interval between cleaning storage systems is lengthened, and crust formation is avoided by eliminating the particles from manure streams. These methods are typically low-cost and low-tech when compared to anaerobic digesters. They do, however, demand more work and time from the maker.

By altering the amount and make-up of manure, changing animal diets can also be utilized as a mitigation strategy. By harmonizing dietary proteins and feed additives, GHG emissions can be reduced. Animals can excrete less nitrogen if they eat less protein. It is also widely known that some supplements, such as tannins, may be able to lower emissions. Tannins can gradually reduce emissions by causing a switch in the excretion of nitrogen from urine to faeces.

**Fertilizer management**

Application of fertilizer to crops used to make animal feed increases nitrous oxide emissions. As a result, mitigation strategies like improving nitrogen use efficiency, breeding and genetically modifying plants using organic fertilizers, routine soil testing, using fertilizers that are state-of-the-art, and planting legumes and grasses together in pasture areas may reduce GHG emissions in the production of feed. The efficiency of nitrogen use can be improved by putting the right amount of nitrogen where the crop can easily get it and at the precise time when it needs the nutrients. A nutrient management strategy may involve routine soil testing, depending on the area and crop, to improve the utilization of nitrogen. Genetic modifications and plant breeding can increase a crop's ability to absorb nitrogen, reducing the requirement for fertilizers.

In order to reduce the deterioration of the fertilizer's and keep the nutrients available to the plant, fertilizer technology has advanced by controlling the release of nutrients from the fertilizers and avoiding nitrification. These modern fertilizers are more expensive than the older methods mentioned above, though. Together, legumes and grasses can significantly lower the amount of synthetic nitrogen required in pasturelands. Because legumes use Rhizobium bacteria to fix nitrogen, less additional nitrogen is required.

## 5. Shifting human dietary trends

The majority of research focuses on reducing GHG emissions from the livestock production sector. However, there hasn't been as much study on the demand side of using livestock products. Reducing meat consumption, as was discussed earlier in this chapter, might significantly reduce greenhouse gas emissions. The livestock sector's beef production has a strong potential for mitigation because it produces the least resource-efficient animal protein and contributes significantly to GHG emissions.

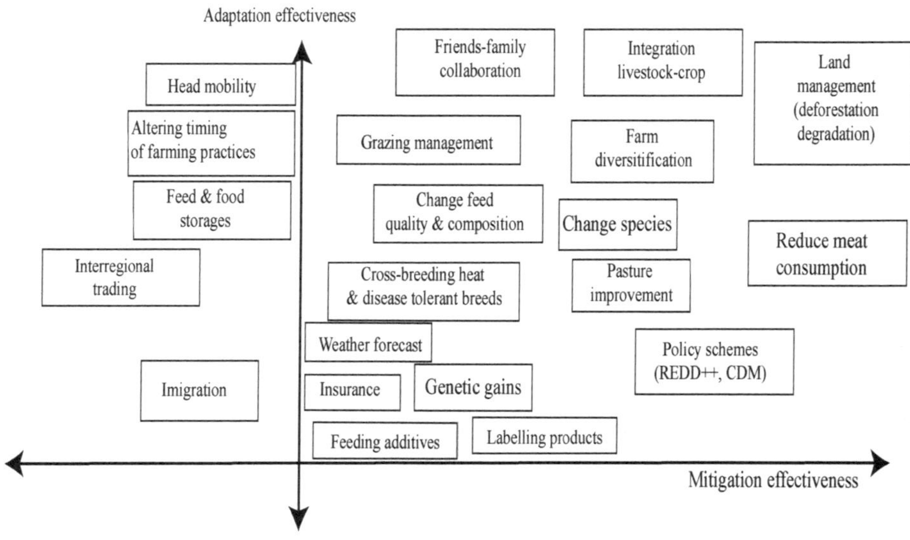


**Fig. 6:** Effectiveness of different adaptations and mitigation options

# 7

# Project Formulation and Evaluation of Various Integrated Livestock Enterprises in Light of Reducing Poverty, Livelihood Diversification, Environmental Sustainability and Resource Conservation

*Lokesh Gautam*

***Project proposal on Integrated Livestock Farming System to Promote Food Security and Livelihood of poor farmers "***

## Why integrated farming?

Integrated farming places a strong emphasis on the fundamental functions of agro-ecosystems, balanced nutrient cycles that are adapted to the demands of the crops, the health and wellbeing of the farm's livestock, and a holistic management strategy that sees the entire farm as one connected system (Kochewad et al. 2017). Family farming, often referred to as integrated farming, provides the opportunity to profitably utilize the farm family's available labor to the fullest extent throughout the year, leading to an increase in income and family contentment. Little dependency on outside supplies and efficient resource recycling on the farm are goals of a good ILFS.

## Project summary

For farmers to earn more money, crop-based agriculture must be diversified to include dairy, goatery, fishing, poultry, duckery, and other enterprises (Ray et al.2012). The farming system places a lot of focus on effectively recycling farm wastes.In an integrated farming system, various farming system components work together to produce a higher overall productivity than the sum of their individual outputs. The efficiency of resource usage is increased when the output from one organization becomes the input for another. Farmers' land holdings are fragmented; therefore it's important to include land-based businesses like fisheries, poultry, apiaries, field crops, and horticulture into the biophysical and socioeconomic conditions of the farmers to increase farming's profitability and dependability (Mahjan et al. 2012).

Nutrition and livelihoods, which can provide low-income tribal farmers with a steady source of revenue to support their way of life, is among the most important emerging sectors. A multidisciplinary holistic strategy known as the integrated farming system method can help small and marginal tribal farmers solve their challenges. The viability and profitability of tribal farmers are seriously threatened by the trend of decreasing land availability per person. In these circumstances, it is appropriate to incorporate land-based businesses such as crop production, dairy, horticultural crops, poultry, and fisheries into the farm with the aim of providing tribal farmers with adequate income and employment and enhancing their standard of living and nutritional security. These tribal farmers used a conventional monoculture agricultural strategy that was experimental, putting an enormous strain on the soil and water resources beyond what they could sustain. The farming system and the sustainability of agriculture production are currently in peril. This shows that the development of an integrated livestock farming system is urgently needed, one in which the many components of the farming system may be linked to boost output and profitability, conserve resources, and protect the environment.

## Integrated livestock based project models (sample models)

### 1. *Fish-poultry based farming system*

It has been suggested to conduct integrated fish farming and poultry farming by taking into account the land that is available to small and marginal farmers in society and member farmers. It will encourage the most efficient use of existing available resources and increase society and farmer member revenue. Since there is a significant need for fish and meat in the neighborhood market, we may take advantage of this need to satisfy clients with dependable service and superior goods. Integrated fish and poultry farming offer the chance to use resources with a minimum of human resources, while also reducing the risk to the business's income and profitability. As we have seen in one industry, the sustainability of agriculture as a source of income for farmers is always in doubt due to natural disasters and market hardship. The cultivation and production of broiler (chicken) would take place on two acres of land, under the management of four persons. In a 400 square meter space, 2000 birds will be grown, and in an 8000 square meter space, 10,000 fingerlings will be stocked. Integrated fish farming is a successful enterprise that may be supported for startup, according to the project's 8-year review. The project's recommendation is supported by the following factors:

## I. Financial analysis

### A) Fish farming

### Assumptions: (e.g. Catla, Rohu etc)

| Particulars | Unit | Value |
|---|---|---|
| Area | $M^2$ | 8000 |
| Pond renovation | Rs. | 150,000 |
| Stocking density of fish | 5000/Per acre | 10,000 |
| Price/ fingerling | Rs. | 2.55 |
| Feed cost /kg | Rs. | 32 |
| Production in tons per year | Tons /year | 5 |
| Production in kgs | Kg | 5,000 |
| | | |
| Total Cost of feed | Rs. | 150,000 |
| Average price /kg | Rs. | 140 |
| Total Revenue | - | 599,930 |
| Seasonal | year | 1 |
| Purchase of Boat, Net, Icebox ( inputs) | - | 200,000 |
| Cost of Other Materials | - | 20,000 |
| Depreciation cost on Fixed assets | % | 5 |
| Interest rate | % | 11 |
| Moratorium | # of year | 1 |
| Repayment Period | -- | 7 |
| Payments Per Year | - | 2 |

### Capital outlay or expenditure

| Particulars | Amount | statements |
|---|---|---|
| **Fixed cost** | | |
| Pond Renovation | 150,000 | 8000 $m^2$ |
| Purchase of Net, Boat, Icebox | 200,000 | Input Purchase |
| Miscellaneous expenses | 21,000 | |
| **Total Fixed Cost** | **371,000** | |
| **Other expenses** | | |
| Hatchlings | 24,999 | Rs. 2.55/Fingerlings |
| Feeding Bags | 150,000 | Rs. 32/Kg bag |
| **Sub-total** | **545,000** | |

## Contribution

| Equity | 20% | 109,000 |
|---|---|---|
| Loan | 80% | 436,000 |
| Total | 100% | 545,000 |

| Particulars/ Years | 1 | 2 | 3 | 4 | 5 | 6 | 7 | 8 |
|---|---|---|---|---|---|---|---|---|
| Total no. of Hatchling | 10,000 | 10,000 | 10,000 | 10,000 | 10,000 | 10,000 | 10,000 | 10,000 |
| Total Cycles assumed per Year | 1 | 1 | 1 | 1 | 1 | 1 | 1 | 1 |
| Total Production in Year (Kg) | 4999.5 | 5259 | 5512 | 5787 | 6077 | 6380 | 6699 | 7035 |
| Price of fish per kg. | 140 | 147 | 154 | 162 | 170 | 179 | 188 | 196 |
| Total Revenue generated | 699,930 | 771,603 | 848,848 | 937,494 | 1,033,090 | 1,142,020 | 1,259,412 | 1,378,860 |

* *It is anticipated that production would rise by 5% annually.*

## Production computation

### Recurring cost

| Years | 1 | | | 2 | 3 | 4 | 5 | 6 | 7 | 8 |
|---|---|---|---|---|---|---|---|---|---|---|
| Particulars | Quantity | Rate | Total | | | | | | | |
| Hatchling | 14,000 | 3 | 35,000 | 36750 | 38588 | 40516 | 42542 | 44669 | 46902 | 49248 |
| Feed | 8,000 | 30 | 240,000 | 252000 | 264600 | 277829 | 291721 | 306307 | 321622 | 337703 |
| Labor | 2 | 8,000 | 192,000 | 201600 | 211679 | 222263 | 233376 | 245045 | 257297 | 270162 |
| | | | 467,000 | 490,350 | 514,867 | 540,611 | 567,608 | 596,021 | 625,821 | 657,113 |

* The cost of labor, feed, and hatching is predicted to increase by 5%.

## Loan repayment

| | | | |
|---|---|---|---|
| | Equity | 109,000 | |
| | Loan | 436,000 | |
| | Total | 545,000 | |
| | Interest | 10.60% | |
| No. of Installments | Principal Balance amount | Principal Equated Half Yearly | Actual Interest |
| 1 | 436,000 | 0 | 23,108.00 |
| 2 | 436,000 | 0 | 23,108.00 |
| 3 | 436,000 | 31,143.00 | 23,108.00 |
| 4 | 404,857 | 31,143.00 | 21,457.42 |
| 5 | 373,714 | 31,143.00 | 19,806.84 |
| 6 | 342,571 | 31,143.00 | 18,156.26 |
| 7 | 311,428 | 31,143.00 | 16,505.68 |
| 8 | 280,285 | 31,143.00 | 14,855.11 |
| 9 | 249,142 | 31,143.00 | 13,204.53 |
| 10 | 217,999 | 31,143.00 | 11,553.95 |
| 11 | 186,856 | 31,143.00 | 9,903.37 |
| 12 | 155,713 | 31,143.00 | 8,252.79 |
| 13 | 124,570 | 31,143.00 | 6,602.21 |
| 14 | 93,427 | 31,143.00 | 4,951.63 |
| 15 | 62,284 | 31,143.00 | 3,301.05 |
| 16 | 31,141 | 31,143.00 | 1,650.47 |
| | **Total** | **436,002.00** | **219,525.31** |
| Payment of Principal amount | 436,002.23 | | |
| Total Interest Paid | 219,525.33 | | |
| Total Paid | 655,527.56 | | |
| Years | 8.00 | | |

## B) Poultry farming (broiler unit)

### Assumptions

| Particulars | Unit | Value |
|---|---|---|
| No of Broiler chicks | Nos | 2,000 |
| Required area ($m^2$) | Sq.Mt. | 400 |
| Price/Hatchling | Rs. | 20 |
| Mortality Rate of chicks | percent | 10% |
| Feed Cost (Bags/Day) | Number of Bags | 3.00 |
| Price /Per Bag | Rs. | 1,300 |
| Cost of feed /Day | Rs. | 3,900 |

| Particulars | Unit | Value |
|---|---|---|
| Rearing Cycle in days | Days | 45 |
| Total Cycles annually | year | 8 |
| Labor charges | 02 Nos. | Rs. 8000/month |
| Electricity charges | | 1,00,000/year |
| Vaccination/Medicines | Rs. | 20,000 |
| Material Costing | Rs. | 50,000 |
| Bird Weight at 45 Days | Kg | 2.15 |
| Meat cost /Kg | Rs. | 70 |
| Profit/Bird (Rs) | Rs. | 10 |
| Depreciation/Year | % | 10% |
| Interest rate | % | 10.6 |
| Moratorium | # of year | 1 |
| Period of Debt Repayment | - | 7 |
| No of Payments anually | | 2 |

## Capital expenditure /contribution

| Particulars/Years | Amount | Remarks |
|---|---|---|
| **Fixed Cost** | | |
| Construction of shed | 200,000 | 400 Sq.Mt |
| Material Costing | 40,000 | Chick, Drinkers etc |
| Miscellaneous Expenses | 20,000 | |
| **Total Fixed amount** | **260,000** | |
| **Other Cost** | | |
| Hatchling Costing | 288,000 | Rs. 18/Hatchling |
| Vaccination | 20,000 | |
| Feeding Bags | 175,500 | 3 Bags/Day |
| **Sub Total** | **1,003,500** | |

## Contribution

| Equity | 20% | 200,700 |
|---|---|---|
| Loan | 80% | 802,800 |
| Total | 100% | 1,003,500 |

## Calculation of production

| Particulars | I | II | III | IV | V | VI | VII | VIII |
|---|---|---|---|---|---|---|---|---|
| Sum of Hatchlings | 2,000 | 2,000 | 2,000 | 2,000 | 2,000 | 2,000 | 2,000 | 2,000 |
| Total Circles (Assumed) | 8 | 8 | 8 | 8 | 8 | 8 | 8 | 8 |
| Average weight/ Chicken | 2.15 | 2.21 | 2.28 | 2.35 | 2.42 | 2.49 | 2.57 | 2.64 |
| Mortality Rate | 10% | 10% | 10% | 10% | 10% | 10% | 10% | 10% |
| Overall Production Per Year (Kgs.) | 30,960 | 31,889 | 32,845 | 33,831 | 34,846 | 35,891 | 36,968 | 38,077 |
| **Sale price of Processed goods** | | | | | | | | |
| Chicken | **70** | 73.5 | 77.18 | 81.0 | 85.09 | 89.34 | 93.81 | 98.50 |
| **Computation of Sales** | | | | | | | | |
| **Overall Sales** | 2,167,200 | 2,343,827 | 2,534,849 | 2,741,439 | 2,964,866 | 3,206,503 | 3,467,833 | 3,750,461 |

**Expected annual increases in production and price are 3% and 5%, respectively.*

## Determination of recurring cost

| S.N | Particulars | I | II | III | IV | V | VI | VII | VIII |
|---|---|---|---|---|---|---|---|---|---|
| | Capital Expenditure | 260000 | 0 | 0 | 0 | 0 | 0 | 0 | 0 |
| | **Recurring Cost** | | | | | | | | |
| 1 | Hatching Cost | 288,000 | 302400 | 317520 | 333396 | 350065.8 | 367569.1 | 385947.5 | 405244.9 |
| 2 | Poultry Feed | 1,404,000 | 1474200 | 1547910 | 1625306 | 1706571 | 1791899 | 1881494 | 1975569 |
| 3 | Medicines | 20,000 | 21000 | 22050 | 23152.5 | 24310.13 | 25525.63 | 26801.91 | 28142.01 |
| 4 | Salary of 2 labours (Rs. 8000/Month) | 192000 | 201600 | 211680 | 222264 | 233377.2 | 245046.1 | 257298.4 | 270163.3 |
| 5 | Electricity charges (Per annum) | 100000 | 105000 | 110250 | 115762.5 | 121550.6 | 127628.2 | 134009.6 | 140710 |
| | Overall Recurring Cost | 2,004,000 | 2,104,200 | 2,209,410 | 2,319,881 | 2,435,875 | 2,557,668 | 2,685,552 | 2,819,829 |

*It is anticipated that there will be a 5% growth per year.

## Repayment schedule

| Equity | 200700 |
|---|---|
| Loan | 802,800 |
| Toal | 1,003,500 |
| Interest | 10.60% |

## 2. Crop- livestock- fishery –Poultry-vermicomposting system

***Project summary***

***Project details (sample model)***

### Assumptions

1. An annual growth in sale prices of Rs. 5 per liter is anticipated.
2. Feed prices are anticipated to rise by Rs. 5 annually.
3. Every year, salaries are anticipated to rise by 5%.
4. The interest rate on term loans is 10% per year.
5. Land investments are anticipated from internal accruals
6. Income taxes are based on individual rates under the 1961 Income Tax Act.
7. Buffalo and other equipment depreciation is computed at 10% on a straight-line basis.

***I Financial details***

| | |
|---|---|
| Total cost of project | 15,00,000.00 lakhs |
| Facilities required | Term Loan |
| Promoters contribution | 1,50,000 |
| Loan from bank | 13,50,000 |
| Moratorium | 6months |
| Break-Even Point (BEP) Fixed Costs ÷ (Revenue per Unit – Variable Cost per) | 62.52% |
| Average DSCR (debt service coverage ratio ) | 1.60 |

***II Project Cost***

| S.No. | Particulars | Amount (lakhs) |
|---|---|---|
| 1. | Cost of animal<br>Species : Buffalo ,breed :Murrah | |
| | 10 buffaloes each @ 10,0000 | 10.0 |
| 2. | Shed cost ,60* 30 sft/ buffalo<br>Total sqft. Required 1800*<br>Cost of construction per sqft.@200 Rs._ | 2.7 |
| 3. | Cost of chicks (indigenous breed e.g kadaknath)<br>100 Rs./chick | 0.03 |
| 4. | Cost of goat<br>10 goats each @ 4000 | 0.4 |

| S.No. | Particulars | Amount (lakhs) |
|---|---|---|
| 5. | Chaff Cutter 3HP | 0.14 |
| 6. | Milking Machine | 0.12 |
| 7. | Bore Well | 0.65 |
| 8. | Motor 3HP | 0.2 |
| 9. | Electrical Wiring | 0.2 |
| 10. | Field Lease | 0.36 |
| 11. | Miscellaneous | 0.2 |
| | **Total cost** | **15.0** |

## Means of Finance: Term Loan

| S.No. | Particulars | Amount (lakhs) | % |
|---|---|---|---|
| 1. | Promoters contribution | 1.5 | |
| 2. | Bank finance | 13.5 | |
| | Total | 15.0 | 100 |

| S.No. | Particulars | Amount (lakhs) | % |
|---|---|---|---|
| 1. | Total working capital | 12,05,200 | 99.058 |

## Yield statement –Milk

| Particulars | 1st year | 2nd Year | 3rd Year | 4th Year | 5th Year |
|---|---|---|---|---|---|
| Total milk installed capacity in lts. (buffalo) | 10.0 | 10.0 | 10.0 | 10.0 | 10.0 |
| No. of buffaloes | 10 | 10 | 10 | 10 | 10 |
| No. of production days in year | 290.0 | 290.0 | 290.0 | 290.0 | 290.0 |
| Total installed capacity | 29000 | 29000 | 31900 | 34800 | 34800 |
| Capacity utilization (%) | 90.0 | 90.0 | 90.0 | 90.0 | 90.0 |
| Actual capacity in lt. | 26100 | 26100 | 28710 | 31320 | 31320 |
| Selling price/lt. | 65 | 65 | 65 | 65 | 70 |
| Total revenue /year | 16,96,500 | 16,96,500 | 18,66,150 | 20,35,800 | 21,92,400 |

## Yield statement –poultry

| Particulars | 1st year | 2nd Year | 3rd Year | 4th Year | 5th Year |
|---|---|---|---|---|---|
| Total installed capacity eggs | 50 | 60 | 70 | 80 | 100 |
| No. of production days in year | 270.0 | 270.0 | 270.0 | 270.0 | 270.0 |
| Total installed capacity | 13,500 | 16,200 | 18,900 | 21,600 | 27000 |
| Selling price/ egg | 10 | 10 | 10 | 10 | 10 |
| Total revenue /year | 1,35000 | 16,2000 | 1,89000 | 21,6000 | 270,000 |

## Yield statement –Meat

| Particulars | 1st year | 2nd Year | 3rd Year | 4th Year | 5th Year |
|---|---|---|---|---|---|
| Total installed capacity kgs | 150 | 150 | 200 | 200 | 250 |
| No. of production in year(batch) | 2 | 2 | 2 | 2 | 2 |
| Total installed capacity | 300 | 300 | 300 | 300 | 300 |
| Selling price/ kg | 700 | 700 | 700 | 750 | 750 |
| Total revenue /year | 1,12,500 | 1,12,500 | 1,50,000 | 1,60,000 | 200,000 |

## Yield statement –Vermi-compost

| Particulars | 1st Year | 2nd Year | 3rd Year | 4th Year | 5th Year |
|---|---|---|---|---|---|
| Sale of vermin compost in kgs | 4000 | 4000 | 4000 | 4000 | 4000 |
| Sale price per kg | 8 | 8 | 8 | 8 | 10 |
| Total revenue | 32,000 | 32000 | 32,000 | 32000 | 40,000 |

## Cost of buffaloes

| Particulars | 1st Year | 2nd Year | 3rd Year | 4th Year | 5th Year |
|---|---|---|---|---|---|
| **A) Feed cost** | | | | | |
| 1.Feed cost /day/buffalo | 310 | 310 | 310 | 360 | 360 |
| 2.No. of buffaloes | 10 | 10 | 11 | 11 | 12 |
| 3.No.of days in a year | 270 | 270 | 270 | 270 | 270 |
| Total feed cost | 8,37,000 | 8,37,000 | 1,069,200 | 1,069,200 | 1,166,400 |

## Cost of chicks

| Particulars | 1st Year | 2nd Year | 3rd Year | 4th Year | 5th Year |
|---|---|---|---|---|---|
| **A) Feed cost** | | | | | |
| 1. Feed cost /year | 110 | 110 | 110 | 110 | 110 |
| 2. No. of days in a year | 300 | 300 | 300 | 300 | 300 |
| Total feed cost | 33,000 | 33,000 | 33,000 | 33,000 | 33,000 |

## Cost of goats

| Particulars | 1st Year | 2nd Year | 3rd Year | 4th Year | 5th Year |
|---|---|---|---|---|---|
| **A) Feed cost** | | | | | |
| 1.Feed cost /year | 210 | 210 | 210 | 210 | 210 |
| 2.No. of days in year | 300 | 300 | 300 | 300 | 300 |
| Total feed cost | 63,000 | 63,000 | 63,000 | 63,000 | 63,000 |
| Particulars | 1st Year | 2nd Year | 3rd Year | 4th Year | 5th Year |
| **A)Earthworms** | | | | | |
| 1.Purchase cost | 5,200 | 5,200 | 5,200 | 5,200 | 5,200 |
| **B)Labor cost** | | | | | |
| 1.Manpower | 3 | 3 | 3 | 3 | 3 |
| 2.Salary/month | 10,000 | 10,000 | 10,000 | 10,000 | 10,000 |
| 3.total salary | 3,60,000 | 3,60,000 | 3,60,000 | 3,60,000 | 3,60,000 |

| Particulars | 1st Year | 2nd Year | 3rd Year | 4th Year | 5th Year |
|---|---|---|---|---|---|
| **C)Medicines /year** | 10,000 | 11,000 | 12,100 | 13,310 | 14,641 |
| **D)Insurance@2% on animal** | - | - | - | - | - |
| **E) Electricity cost / year** | 20,000 | 22,000 | 24,200 | 26,620 | 29,282 |

## Projected profitability statement

| | Projected | Projected | Projected | Projected | Projected |
|---|---|---|---|---|---|
| **Particulars** | **1st Year** | **2nd Year** | **3rd Year** | **4th Year** | **5th Year** |
| **Income** | | | | | |
| Sales Revenue | 19,76,000 | 17,28,500 | 18,98,150 | 20,67,800 | 22,32,400 |
| Other Income | - | - | - | - | - |
| **Total** | **19,76,000** | **17,28,500** | **18,98,150** | **20,67,800** | **22,32,400** |
| **Expenditure** | | | | | |
| Feed Cost | 9,05,200 | 8,15,200 | 8,96,200 | 10,44,700 | 11,39,200 |
| Salaries & Wages | 3,60,000 | 3,60,000 | 3,60,000 | 3,60,000 | 4,32,000 |
| Medicine Cost | 10,000 | 11,000 | 12,100 | 13,310 | 14,641 |
| Electricity Charges | 20,000 | 22,000 | 24,200 | 26,620 | 29,282 |
| Miscellaneous expenses | - | - | - | - | - |
| Finance Charges | 1,78,875 | 95,625 | 68,625 | 41,625 | 14,625 |
| Depreciation | 1,50,000 | 1,50,000 | 1,50,000 | 1,50,000 | 1,50,000 |
| **Profit Before Tax** | 3,51,925 | 2,74,675 | 3,87,025 | 4,31,545 | 4,52,652 |
| Provision for Tax | - | | - | 1,29,464 | 1,35,796 |
| **Profit After Tax** | **3,51,925** | **2,74,675** | **3,87,025** | **3,02,082** | **3,16,856** |
| **Net Profit Ratio** | **17.81%** | **15.89%** | **20.39%** | **14.61%** | **14.19%** |

## Ratio of Debt Service Coverage (DSCR)

| | Projected | Projected | Projected | Projected | Projected |
|---|---|---|---|---|---|
| **Particulars** | **1st Year** | **2nd Year** | **3rd Year** | **4th Year** | **5th Year** |
| Profit After tax | 3,51,925 | 2,74,675 | 3,87,025 | 3,02,082 | 3,16,856 |
| Depreciation | 1,50,000 | 1,50,000 | 1,50,000 | 1,50,000 | 1,50,000 |
| Term loan interest | 1,78,875 | 95,625 | 68,625 | 41,625 | 14,625 |
| **Total** | **6,80,800** | **5,20,300** | **6,05,650** | **4,93,707** | **4,81,481** |
| **Payment Obligation** | | | | | |
| TL Installments | 2,70,000 | 2,70,000 | 2,70,000 | 2,70,000 | 2,70,000 |
| **Total** | **4,48,875** | **3,65,625** | **3,38,625** | **3,11,625** | **2,84,625** |
| **DSCR** | **1.52** | **1.42** | **1.79** | **1.58** | **1.69** |
| **Average DSCR** | **1.60** | - | - | - | - |

## Break Even Point (BEP)

| Particulars | Projected 1st Year | Projected 2nd Year | Projected 3rd Year | Projected 4th Year | Projected 5th Year |
|---|---|---|---|---|---|
| Revenue | 19,76,000 | 17,28,500 | 18,98,150 | 20,67,800 | 22,32,400 |
| **Variable Costs** | | | | | |
| Feed Cost | 9,05,200 | 8,15,200 | 8,96,200 | 10,44,700 | 11,39,200 |
| Medicine Cost | 10,000 | 11,000 | 12,100 | 13,310 | 14,641 |
| **Total** | **9,15,200** | **8,26,200** | **9,08,300** | **10,58,010** | **11,53,841** |
| **Contribution** | **10,60,800** | **9,02,300** | **9,89,850** | **10,09,790** | **10,78,559** |
| **Fixed Costs** | | | | | |
| Salaries | 3,60,000 | 3,60,000 | 3,60,000 | 3,60,000 | 4,32,000 |
| Electricity Charges | 20,000 | 22,000 | 24,200 | 26,620 | 29,282 |
| Interest | 1,78,875 | 95,625 | 68,625 | 41,625 | 14,625 |
| Depreciation | 1,50,000 | 1,50,000 | 1,50,000 | 1,50,000 | 1,50,000 |
| **Total** | **7,08,875** | **6,27,625** | **6,02,825** | **5,78,245** | **6,25,907** |
| **Break-even Point** | **66.82%** | **69.56%** | **60.90%** | **57.26%** | **58.03%** |
| **Break even Sales** | **13,20,453** | **12,02,316** | **11,55,986** | **11,84,103** | **12,95,501** |
| **Margin of Safety Sales** | **6,55,547** | **5,26,184** | **7,42,164** | **8,83,697** | **9,36,899** |
| **Average BEP** | **62.52%** | | | | |

1. Integrated farming system model of Field Crop + Horticultural crops +Bee keeping + Goat Farming + Broiler Poultry +Fodder + Mushroom + Vermicomposting

## 1. Project summary

The livelihood of small and poor farmers depends on Agriculture, livestock, and vegetable cultivation. The majority of farmers have small and marginal land holdings, inadequate resources, and poor livestock management. Consequently they are getting low income per capita. Looking to the climate variations the productivity of crops is decreasing due to reliance upon a few crops in combination with crops like Pearl-millet, sesame, Green gram, Black Gram, mustard, gram and wheat etc. along with poor livestock husbandry practices. This Integrated Farming System component is best suited for minimizing the risk, increasing production and profit along with improving the utilization of organic waste and crop residue. The suggested IFS model will raise awareness among farmers and give them the information, inspiration, and skills they need to begin a systematic plan on their fields for better resource usage, which will lead to higher per-capita income and sustainable agriculture. Through a combination of crop, horticulture, livestock, beekeeping, and other forms of agriculture, they can also reduce risk while increasing production and profit and enhancing the utilization of organic wastes and crop residues. Finally, they could guarantee their ability to support themselves, make the best use of available resources, maintain soil fertility, and stop soil degradation.

## 2. Component of IFS Model (1.0 ha)

***Field Crop + Horticultural crops +Bee keeping + Goat Farming + Broiler Poultry +Fodder +Mushroom + Vermicomposting***

**I. Integration of cropping**

Crop – Pearl-millet, pigeon-pea, Soybean, cluster bean, Green gram, Black gram, Wheat, Gram & mustard.

II. Integration of Horticulture

(a) **Vegetable cultivation**: on mulching, drip irrigation (Tomato, chilli,potato, cucumber ,onion etc)

(b) **Fruits:** High density orchids, Plantation of apples, guava, oranges etc.

(c) **Floriculture:** Marigold, rose, sunflower etc.

**III. Goatery**: Sirohi , Jamunapari,Barbari etc.

**IV. Poultry** : Commercial Broiler poultry birds

**V. Beekeeping** : Apis melifera (Honey production & pollination)

**VI. Vermicomposting**: Eisenia foetida (worms and compost)

**VII. Mushroom**: Oster and Button

VIII. Fodder & Azola production for goatry

***Project details***

| S. No. | Item | Area ($m^2$) | No/Unit |
|---|---|---|---|
| I | RCT in Pearlmillet, clusterbean, Soybean, Pigeon pea, Black gram, Green Gram, Wheat, Gram | 3000 | 01 |
| II (a) | Tomato, Chili, Cucumber, brinjal, Potato, Onion etc. (Mulching, net house, Drip system) | 1000 | 01 |
| II (b) | High density Orchard – Ber. Guava, Drumstick, Aonla, lime etc. | 2000 | 01 |
| II (c ) | Floriculture | 1000 | 01 |
| III | Goat | 900 | 01 |
| IV | Beekeeping | 1400 | 01 |
| V | Broiler Poultry | 300 | 01 |
| VI | Vermicomposting | 200 | 01 |
| VII | Mushroom | 200 | 01 |
| | TOTAL | 10000 | 09 |

## *Financial details* (budget analysis)

| S.No. | Particulars | Specifications | No. ofunits | Amountrequired (Rs. In lakhs) |
|---|---|---|---|---|
| I | RCT in Pearlmillet, clusterbean, Soybean, Pigeon pea, Black gram, Green Gram, Wheat, Gram | 0.3ha | 01 | 0.25 |
| II | High density orchards with drip irrigation | 0.2 ha | 01 | 1.0 |
| III | Tomato, Chili, Cucumber, brinjal, Potato, Onion etc. (Mulching, net house, Drip system) | 0.1ha | 01 | 1.0 |
| IV | Floriculture | 0.1ha | 01 | 0.25 |
| V | Goatery | | | |
| | Shed (@ Rs 600/Sq feet) | 15' x 20' | 01 | 2.0 |
| | Goats | Barbari/ Jamunapari / Sirohi | 10 | 1.0 |
| | Miscellaneous (Feed + Feeders + Waterers + Medicine) | | | 0.20 |
| VI | broiler poultry unit (For 1000 birds) | 20' x 50' | 01 | 2.0 |
| VII | Bee keeping (100 bee colonies) | 100 bee box with colony) | 01 | 4.0 |
| VIII | Vermicomposting | 0.02ha | 01 | 0.50 |
| IX | Renovation of existing mushroom unit | - | 01 | 0.50 |
| X | Miscellaneous (Implements & tools, Staking material, budding & graftingmaterials etc.) | - | - | 0.30 |
| **Total - Thirteen lakh Rupees only** | | | | **13.0** |

## Expected outcome (After 2 years)

| Components wise production | Area/No (ha) | Gross return (Rs. In lakhs) |
|---|---|---|
| Agriculture produce | 0.300 | 1.50 |
| Horticulture produce | 0.400 | 2.00 |
| Goat production | 0.090 | 4.0 |
| Poultry birds | 0.030 | 1.30 |
| Bee keeping | 0.140 | 4.00 |
| Vermicomposting | 0.020 | 0.60 |
| Mushroom | 0.020 | 0.40 |
| TOTAL | 1.000 | 13.80 |

# Bibliography


Ahmadi, B.V., Moran, D., Barnes, A.P., Baret, P.V., 2015. Comparing decision-support systems in adopting sustainable intensification criteria. *Frontier Genetics*. 6, 1–5.

Alam, M.R., Sarker, R.I., Hossain M.D. and Islam, M.S. (2000).Contribution of livestock to small farms in Bangladesh. *Asian Australasian Journal of Animal Science*. 13:339-342

Amandeep Singh (2018).https://www.pashudhanpraharee.com/role-of-livestock-in-indian-economy/ assessed on 12.12.2022.

Atherstone, C., Grace, D., Lindahl, J., Kang'ethe, E.K., Nelson, F.( 2016). Assessing the impact of aflatoxin consumption on animal health and productivity. *African Jounal of Food Agriculture and Nutrition Development*. 16, 10949–10966.

Beauchemin, K.A., McAllister, T.A., McGinn, S.M. (2009). Dietary mitigation of enteric methane from cattle. CAB reviews: perspectives in agriculture, veterinary science. *Nutrition Natural Resource*. 4 (35), 1–8.

Bellarby, J., Tirado, R., Leip, A., Weiss, F., Lesschen, J.P., Smith, P. (2013). Livestock greenhouse gas emissions and mitigation potential in Europe. *Global. Change Biology*. 19, 3–18.

Behera, U. K., Jha, K. P. and Mahapatra, I.C. (2004). Integrated management ofavailable resources of the small and marginal farmers for generation of income and employment in eastern India. *Crop Research,* 27: 83-89.

Boadi, D., Benchaar, C., Chiquette, J., Massé, D., 2004. Mitigation strategies to reduce enteric methane emissions from dairy cows: update review. *Canadian Journal of Animal Science*. 84, 319–335.

Bruinsma, J., 2003. World Agriculture: Towards 2015/2030: An FAO Perspective. *Earth scan*, London.

Casey, K.D., Bicudo, J.R., Schmidt, D.R., Singh, A., Gay, S.W., Gates, R.S., Jacobson, L.D., Hoff, S.J., (2006).Air quality and emissions from livestock and poultry production/waste management systems. In Animal Agriculture and the Environment: National Center for Manure and Waste Management White Papers. American Society of Agricultural and Biological Engineers, St. Joseph, Mich, p. 40.

Chhabra, A., Manjunath, K.R., Panigrahy, S., Parihar, J.S., 2013 Greenhouse gas emissions from Indian livestock. *Climatic Change* 117, 329–344.

Chapman, S.C., Chakraborty, S., Dreccer, M.F., Howden, S.M., 2012. Plant adaptation to climate change: opportunities and priorities in breeding. *Crop Pasture Science*. 63, 251–268.

Dayanandan, R. ( 2011). Production and marketing efficiency of dairy farms in highland of Ethiopia–an economic analysis. International Journal of Enterpise Computer. Bus System.

Dash, S. (2017).Contribution of Livestock Sector to Indian Economy. *Indian Journal of Research,* 6:890-891.

Department of Animal Husbandry, Dairying and Fisheries. Government of India, 20th Livestock Census; 2019.accessed on 12.12.2022.

Devendra, C. and Pezo, D. (2002). Improvement of crop animal systems in rainfed agriculture to food security and livelihoods in south East Asia. In; Proceedings International symposium onsustaining food security and managing natural resources in South East Asia, Einselen Foundation, Ulm, Germany and Chiang Mai 1 University, Chiang Mai. pp. 129-131.

Dickie, A., Streck, C., Roe, S., Zurek, M., Haupt, F., Dolginow, A. (2014). Strategies for mitigating climate change in agriculture: Abridged report. Climate focus and california environmental associates, prifadred with the support of the climate and land use Alliance. Report and supplementary materials available at: <www.agriculturalmitigation.org>.

Dorward, A., Chirwa, E., 2014. The rehabilitation of agricultural input subsidies? IIED Working Paper: Food and Agriculture. IIED, London.

DSI MSU, 2015.Decision support and informatics. Michigan State University. <http://dsiweb.cse.msu.edu/>.

FAO (1989). Farming Systems Development: Concept, Methods, Applications, Food and Agriculture Organization of the United Nations, Rome.

FAO (Food and Agriculture Organization of the United Nations), (2009a). Global agriculture towards 2050. High Level Expert Forum Issues Paper. FAO, Rome.

FAO (Food and Agriculture Organization of the United Nations), (2007). The state of the world's animal genetic resources for food and agriculture: in brief, edited by Barbara Rischkowsky & Dafydd Pilling, Rome.

FAO (Food and Agriculture Organization of the United Nations), (2017). GAEZ - Global Agro-Ecological Zones. <http://www.fao.org/nr/gaez/en/> accessed on12.12.2022.

FAO (Food and Agriculture Organization of the United Nations), (1996). Agro-Ecological Zoning Guidelines. Rome. FAO (Food and Agriculture Organization of the United Nations), 1996. Agro-Ecological Zoning Guidelines. Rome.

FAO (Food and Agriculture Organization of the United Nations), 2013. Climate-smart agriculture: Sourcebook. FAO, Rome. <http://www.fao.org/3/a-i3325e.pdf>.

Garforth, C., 2015. Livestock keepers' reasons for doing and not doing things which governments, vets and scientists would like them to do. Zoonoses Public Health 62, 29–38

Gerber, P.J., Steinfeld, H., Henderson, B., Mottet, A., Opio, C., Dijkman, J., Falcucci, A., Tempio, G., (2013). Tackling Climate Change through Livestock: A Global Assessment of Emissions and Mitigation Opportunities. FAO, Rome.

Ghosh, S. & Klass, D.L. (1978), Process Biochemistry. pg 13, 15.

Godi, N.Y., Zhengwuvi, L.B., Abdulkadir,S. and Kamtu, P. (2013). Effect of cow dungvariety on biogas production. *Journal of Mechanical Engineering Research,* 5:1-4

Grace, D., Gilbert, J., Randolph, T., Kang'ethe, E., 2012a. The multiple burdens of zoonotic disease and an Ecohealth approach to their assessment. Trop. Anim. Health Prod. 44, S67–S73.

Hatfield, J.L., Boote, K., Fay, P., Hahn, L., Izaurralde, C., Kimball, B.A., Mader, T., Morgan, J., Ort, D., Polley, W., Thomson, A., Wolfe, D. (2008). Agriculture, in: Walsh, M., The effects of climate change on agriculture, land resources, water resources, and biodiversity in the United States.A Report by the U.S. Climate Change Science Program and the Subcommittee on Global Change Research. Washington, DC., USA, pp. 362.

Hatfield, J.L., Prueger, J.H. (2011). Agro ecology: implications for plant response to climate change. In: Yadav, S.S., Redden, R.J., Hatfield, J.L., Lotze-Campen, H., Hall, A.E. (Eds.), Crop Adaptation to Climate Change. Wiley-Blackwell, Chichester, UK, pp. 27–43.

Herrero, M., Thornton, P.K., Notenbaert, A., Msangi, S., Wood, S., Kruska, R., Dixon, J., Bossio, D., van de Steeg, J., Ade Freeman, H., Li, X., ParthasarathyRao, P.,( 2012). Drivers of Change in Crop–Livestock Systems and Their Potential Impacts on Agro-Ecosystems Services and Human Wellbeing to 2030: A Study Commissioned by the CGIAR Systemwide Livestock Program. *International Livestock Research Institute, Nairobi, Kenya.*

Herrero, M., Havlik, P., Valin, H., Notenbaert, A., Rufino, M.C., Thornton, P.K., Blummel, M., Weiss, F., Grace, D., Obersteiner, M.(2013b). Biomass use, production, feed efficiencies, and greenhouse gas emissions from global livestock systems. PNAS 110, 20888–20893

Hoffmann, I., (2010). Climate change and the characterization, breeding and conservation of animal genetic resources. *Animal Genetics*. 41, 32–46

IFAD (International Fund for Agricultural Development), (2010). Livestock and climate change. <http://www.ifad.org/lrkm/events/cops/papers/climate.pdf>.

IPCC (Intergovernmental Panel on Climate Change), (1997). IPCC/OECD/IEA Program on national greenhouse gas inventories.Intergovernmental panel on climate change. <http://www.ipccnggip.iges.or.jp/public/mtdocs/pdfiles/rockhamp.pdf

PCC (Intergovernmental Panel on Climate Change), (2014). Climate Change 2014: impacts, adaptation, and vulnerability. part A: global and sectorial aspects Contribution of Working Group II to the Fifth Assessment Report of the Intergovernmental Panel on Climate Change. Cambridge University Press, Cambridge, United Kingdom and New York, NY, USA, p. 1132.

Jayanthi, C., Rangasamy, A. and Chinnusamy, C. (2000). Water budgeting forcomponents in lowland integrated farmingsystems. *Agricultural Journal*, 87:411-416.

Karl, T.R., Melillo, J.M., Peterson, T.C., 2009. Global Climate Change Impacts in the United States. U.S. Global Change Research Programme. CambridgeUniversity Press.

Karl. L., E, Y.O., Genova, R.C., Girma, B., Kissel, E.S., Levy, A.N., MacCracken, S., Mastrandrea, P.R., White, L.L.(2014). Contribution of Working Group II to the Fifth Assessment Report of the Intergovernmental Panel on Climate Change. Cambridge University Press, Cambridge, United Kingdom and New York, NY, USA, p. 1132.

Klapwijk, C.J., Van Wijk, M.T., Rosenstock, T.S., Van Asten, P.J.A., Thornton, P.K., Giller, K.E., 2014. Analysis of trade-offs in agricultural systems: current status and way forward. *Current Opinion in Environmental Sustainability* 6, 110–115.

Kristjanson, P., Waters-Bayer, A., Johnson, N., Tipilda, A., Njuki, J., Baltenweck, I., Grace, D., Macmillan, S., 2014. Livestock and women's livelihoods. In: Quisumbing, A., Meinzen-Dick, R., Raney, T., Croppenstedt, A., Behrman, J., Peterman, A. (Eds.), Gender in Agriculture: Closing the Knowledge Gap. *Food and Agricluture Organization of the United Nations*, Rome, Italy.

Martin, C., Morgavi, D.P., Doreau, M., (2010). Methane mitigation in ruminants: from microbe to the farm scale. *Animal* 4 (3), 351–365.

McDermott, J.J., Staal, S.J., Freeman, H.A., Herrero, M., Van De Steeg, J.A., (2010).Sustaining intensification of smallholder livestock systems in the tropics. *Livestock Science*, 130, 95–109.

Moulik, T.K. (1990), India institute of management, Ahmedabad, In: International Conference on Biogas.

Nardone, A., Ronchi, B., Lacetera, N., Ranieri, M.S., Bernabucci, U.(2010). Effects of climate change on animal production and sustainability of livestock systems. *Livestock Science*, 130, 57–69.

Nirmala, G.,Ramana, D.B.V. andVenkateswarlu, B. (2012). Women and Scientific Livestock Management: Improving Capabilities through Participatory Action Research in Semi -Arid Areas of South India. *APCBEE Procedia* 4:152 – 157.

O'Mara, F.P. (2012).The role of grasslands in food security and climate change. *Annals of Botany*. 110, 1263–1270

Panke, S.K., Kadam, R.P. and Nakhate, C.S., (2010). Integrated Farming System for suatainable rural livelihood security. In: 22nd national seminar on "Role of Extension in Integrated Farming Systems for sustainable rural livelihood, 9th -10th Dec, Maharastra, (pp. 33-35).

Price, E.C. & Cheremisinoff, P.N. (1981). In:*Biogas: Production and Utilization.* Ann Arbor Science Publishers, Collingwood, Michigen. pp 1–10.

Ramana, D.B.V., Reddy, N.N., Rao, G. R. (2011). Hortipastoral systems for ram lamb production in rain fed areas. *Annals of Biological Research,* 2:150.

Ramaswamy, N.S. (1998). Draught animal welfare. *Applied Animal Behaviour Science*.59: 73-84.

Rana SS 2015. Recent Advances in Integrated Farming Systems. Department of Agronomy, College of Agriculture, CSK Himachal Pradesh Krishi Vishvavidyalaya, Palampur, 204 pages.

Ray, M., Samanta, B., Haldar, P., Chatterjee,S. and Khan, D.K. (2012). AgriculturePractices and Its Association with Livestock in Hilly Areas of West Bengal. *Indian Journal of Hill Farming,* 25:53-57

Renaudeau, D., Collin, A., Yahav, S., De Basilio, V., Gourdine, J.L., Collier, R.J., 2012. Adaptation to hot climate and strategies to alleviate heat stress in livestock production. Animal 6 (05), 707–728.

Rojas M.D., Nejadashmi A.P., Harrigan T., Sean A. and Woznicki (2017). Climate change and Livestock: Impacts ,Adaptation and Mitigation. *Climate Risk Management* 16:147-163.

Rubin, D., Tezera, S., Caldwell, L., 2010. A calf, a house, a business of one's own: microcredit, asset accumulation, and economic empowerment in GL CRSP projects in Ethiopia and Ghana. Global Livestock CRSP.

Sahoo, U.K. and Singh, S.L. (2015). Integrated Fish-Pig and Fish-Poultry Farming in East Kalcho, Saiha District of Mizoram, North-East India: An Economic Analysis. *International Journal of Agriculture and Forestry,* 5: 281-286.

Senthilvel, T., Latha, K.R. and Gopalasamy,N. (1998). Farming system approach for sustainable yield and income under rainfed vertisols. *Madras Agriculture Journal*, 55: 65-67

Smith, A., Snapp, S., Chikowo, R., Thorne, P., Bekunda, M., Glover, J., 2017. Measuring sustainable intensification in smallholder agroecosystems: a review. Glob. Food Secur. 12, 127–138.

Steinfeld, H., Gerber, P., Wassenaar, T., Castel, V., Rosales, M., Haan, C.(2006). Livestock's Long Shadow: Environmental Issues and Options. FAO, Rome.

Stuart K, Elizabeth S, Niab; Christopher S. (2019) .Achieving sustainable intensification by integrating livestock into arable systems opportunities and impacts, final report Game And Wildlife Conservation Trust,Allerton Project; and,Niki Rust, School Of Natural and Environmental Sciences, Newcastle University .

Swingland, I.A.(2001). Biodiversity, definition of. *Encyclopedia of Biodiversity*, 1: 377–391.

Takahashi, K., Ikegami, M., Sheahan, M., Barrett, C.B.(2016). Experimental evidence on the drivers of index-based livestock insurance demand in Southern Ethiopia. *World Development* 78, 324–340.

Theriault, V., Smale, M., Haider, H., 2017. How does gender affect sustainable intensification of cereal production in the West African Sahel? Evidence from Burkina Faso. *World Development*. 92, 177–191.

Thornton, P.K., Van de Steeg, J., Notenbaert, A., Herrrero, M.(2009). The impacts of climate change on livestock and livestock systems in developing countries: A review of what we know and what we need to know. *Agricultural System* 101, 113–127.

Thornton, P.K., Herrero, M.(2010). The Inter-linkages between rapid growth in livestock production, climate change, and the impacts on water resources, land use, and deforestation. World Bank Policy Research Working Paper, WPS 5178. World Bank, Washington, DC

Thornton, P.K., Boone, R.B., Ramirez-Villegas J.(2015). Climate change impacts on livestock. CGIAR Resrach program on Climate Change, Agriculture and Food Security (CCAFS), Working Paper No. 120.

Tripathi, S.C., and Rathi, R.C. (2011). Livestock farming system module for hills. In: Souvenir. National symposium on technological interventions for sustainable agriculture, 3rd - 5th May, GBPUAT, hill campus, Ranichuri, (pp. 103 -104).

UNFCCC (United Nations Framework Convention on Climate Change) (1998). Kyoto protocol to the United Nations framework convention on climate change adopted at COP3 in Kyoto, Japan, on 11 December 1997. <http://unfccc.int/resource/docs/convkp/kpeng.pdf>.

UNEP (United Nations Environment Programme), (2012). Global environment outlook 5: Chapter 5. <http://www.unep.org/geo/pdfs/geo5/GEO5_report_C5. pdf>.

USDA (United States Department of Agriculture), (2013). Climate Change and Agriculture in the United States: Effects and Adaptation. USDA technical bulletin, Washington, DC. http://www.usda.gov/oce/climate_change/effects_2012/CC%20and%20Agriculture%20 Report%20%2802-04-2013%29b.pdf.

Venkatadri, S., Swaroopa Rani, K. and Raghunadha Reddy, G. (2008). A study on improvement in rural livelihoods through dairy farming. Centre for Self Employment and Rural Enterprises. National Institute of Rural Development, Rajendranagar,Hyderabad – 500 030.

WEC (World Energy Council), (2015).World Energy Issues Monitor. <http://www.worldenergy.org/wp-content/uploads/2015/01/2015-World-Energy-Issues Monitor.pdf >.

White, N., Sutherst, R.W., Hall, N., Whish-Wilson, P.(2003). The vulnerability of the Australian beef industry to impacts of the cattle tick (Boophilus microplus) under climate change. *Climatic Change*. 61, 157–190.